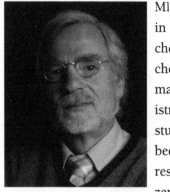

Ml[...] in 1949, and has a doctorate in chemistry. He has worked in the chemical industry as well as pharmaceuticals, and has taught chemistry and biology to secondary school students. For the past 15 years he has been managing director of a cancer research institute in Arlesheim, Switzerland. Since the publication of this book in German, he has embarked on an ever-increasing schedule of lectures and a lively correspondence with numerous individuals.

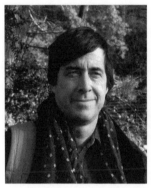

THOMAS STÖCKLI was born in 1951. He has worked as a freelance journalist, a teacher at middle school level, and a lecturer on teacher training and educational research. For the past 25 years he has been intensively concerned with spiritual questions and personal development, and has authored many articles and books on these subjects. He is currently endeavouring to link spiritual ideas with scientific thought, while conversely working against dogmatism in science.

LIFE FROM LIGHT

LIFE FROM LIGHT

IS IT POSSIBLE TO LIVE WITHOUT FOOD?

A SCIENTIST REPORTS ON HIS EXPERIENCES

Michael Werner and Thomas Stöckli

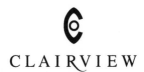

CLAIRVIEW

Translated by J. Collis, member of the Chartered Institute of Linguists

Clairview Books
Hillside House, The Square
Forest Row, RH18 5ES

www.clairviewbooks.com

Published by Clairview 2007
Reprinted 2007

Originally published in German under the title *Leben durch Lichtnahrung*
by AT Verlag, Baden and Munich, 2005

Photos on pages 142, 143, 149 © M. Werner; pages i and 62 © C J. Buess

*The translator is grateful for help with the medical terminology in this book to
Anna Meuss, Fellow of the Chartered Institute of Linguists and Member of the
Society of Authors*

*The Publishers thank Johannes Surkamp for the partial use of his translation of
an article from* Das Goetheanum *(Nr 34-5/2002) that first appeared in
English in* New View *magazine*

A catalogue record for this book is available from the British Library

ISBN 978 1905570 05 8

Cover by Andrew Morgan Design
Typeset by DP Photosetting, Neath, West Glamorgan
Printed and bound by Cromwell Press Limited, Trowbridge, Wiltshire

CONTENTS

PUBLISHER'S NOTE

An important and unambiguous statement

This work is intended first and foremost as a source of information and documentation. It is in no way intended as a recommendation for attempting to receive nourishment from light as an alternative to eating food. Halting consumption of food and drink, for any duration of time, could lead to critical health consequences. Any significant change in diet should be made only after consultation with a medical doctor or a suitably qualified health practitioner.

The publisher and authors do not accept liability for any harm arising either directly or indirectly in connection with the information published here.

Foreword

by Jakob Bösch, MD

Therese Neumann, born at Konnersreuth, Southern Germany, in 1898, stopped eating and drinking before she reached her thirtieth year. Thereafter she consumed only 'one eighth of a small Host [the wafer given at Mass] and about 3 cubic centimetres of water daily [to help her swallow the Host]'. Otherwise she declined any food or drink for 35 years until her death.* Since she also bore the stigmata (wounds resembling those of Christ in hands, feet and side) she soon caused a considerable stir among the general public. This persuaded the Bishop of Regensburg to have her kept under strict observation which included supervision of her visitors. For example, during a 3-week observation period in 1927, four nuns of impeccably reliable character were sworn to keep an uninterrupted watch over her, two at a time, without letting her out of their sight for one second. They were permitted to use only a damp cloth to 'wash' Therese, and no food or drink was allowed in her room. The four nuns stated under oath that the woman under observation had taken neither food nor drink during the course of the 3 weeks apart from the crumb of the Host and the three cubic centimetres of water already mentioned.

At the beginning of the observation period Therese Neumann weighed 55 kilos; on the first Friday, when the stigmata bled, she lost 4 kilos; during the ensuing week her weight rose again to 54

---

*J. Steiner, 1977. (See Bibliography for full references.)

kilos even though she had taken no liquid or food. The same sequence occurred during the second week, and at the end of the observation period she once again weighed 55 kilos.

Medical supervision and assessment was carried out not only by a senior public health official but also by a medical professor from the University of Erlangen, a Protestant, who published the results in the *Münchener Medizinische Wochenschrift.** Fraud was not counted as a plausible explanation either for the abstention from food or for the bleeding of the stigmata.†

The ability to think critically was not born with the twentieth century. In earlier times, too, negation of truth arising out of religious fanaticism was known to persuade some to overlook fraud and deception. After a successful career as a farmer, officer and politician, the national saint of Switzerland, Nicholas von der Flüe (1417–1487), usually known as Brother Klaus, left his family and farm at the age of 50. Having undergone a profound mystical experience, he proceeded to live for a further 20 years until his death without eating or drinking. But even in those days the phenomenon of living without food was not accepted unquestioningly. Although Nicholas was later made a saint, in his day, long before our own materialistic age, many of his contemporaries reacted with scepticism to any talk of his living without food. So a number of young men were contracted to seal off the entrance to the ravine where his hermitage was located for a month in order to prevent any clandestine smuggling in of food and drink, especially during the night. Nevertheless, various well-known personages still held to their scepticism. An emissary of the Bishop of Constance wanted to take matters into his own hands and convict Nicholas of fraud by forcing him to

---

* No. 46, 1927.
† J. Steiner, 1977.

eat. And in order to obey his spiritual superior the pious man of God did indeed endeavour to eat. But having lived without food for so long, his body had changed and the attempt ended in a fiasco and near catastrophe, so that the cleric from Constance had to withdraw without having achieved his goal. Whether he changed his mind is not recorded.* On the other hand, however, history does record the exposure of a number of fraudulent claims regarding living without food.†

Today, scientists whose training has been cast in the traditional mould still feel annoyed and provoked by cases in which food, and especially liquids, have been refused for long periods, seeing them either as a deception or as irresponsible dicing with a person's health. Perhaps this is the most likely reason why such a highly interesting phenomenon has never been properly researched. Yet biophysicists today confirm that electromagnetic radiation accounts for three quarters of the energy supplied and given off in humans and that quantitatively the acquisition of energy via food plays only a small part.‡ We have known at the latest since the development of the quantum theory that light and matter are different states of the same thing. And we have known since the discovery of photosynthesis that sunlight can produce starch, i.e. solid matter or foodstuffs, out of CO_2 and H_2O, though to this day this process is still not scientifically understood in every detail. If we further add the fact that science has proved absolutely that the human spirit can influence living as well as inanimate matter,§ then it should not be too difficult to regard lengthy abstinence from food and liquid intake as being possible in principle. This precondition must

---

* Hemleben, 1977.
† Vandereycken, 1992.
‡ Warnke, 1997.
§ Jahn, 1996.

surely be met if serious researchers are to embark on a close scrutiny of the processes involved in abstinence from food and liquid intake.

The experiment described in this book (see Chapter 4) which was conducted with Michael Werner at a Swiss university hospital will, it is hoped, have pushed open the door to a field that will lead to an as yet incalculable number of new scientific findings. All those who participated deserve to be thanked for their open-mindedness, their courage and their persistence. To obtain the necessary permissions from the ethics commission, the administration and other bodies presented an obstacle course of unprecedented proportions, for if anything had indeed gone wrong, those responsible would have been roundly condemned.

Ellen Greve, alias Jasmuheen, from Australia, the founder of the so-called 21-day process,* herself had to endure the wrath of the scientific community. Apart from being branded a fraud, she also had to submit to various weighty psychiatric diagnoses which, however, left her reputation largely intact. Especially after reports of a death in New Zealand that had occurred during the course of one person's practice of the 21-day process, the media and the medical profession went wild. However, whereas prior to this some individuals may have gone about this type of 'fasting' too carelessly, perhaps those media reports actually did lead to more responsible ways of handling the process that enables people to begin 'living on light'. Anyway, concern about the few deaths that may have occurred among what are presumed to be tens of thousands who have practised the 21-day process is unlikely to be the real reason for the indignation

---

*Jasmuheen, 1998. The 'transition' process to 'living on light'. See further on pages 77–84.

expressed; otherwise the same degree of indignation should surely also be directed towards the far greater proportion of deaths and serious injuries resulting from extreme sporting practices of one kind or another. Moreover, inappropriate diets involving the intake of too much or too little food and liquids lead to death in tens of thousands or even millions of cases without arousing anything like the same degree of indignation. So one cannot help suspecting that the real reason for the protests by both media and medical experts with regard to living on light boils down to the fact that such a way of life does not conform to prevailing views about the world.

After it became known that I, too, had carried out the 21-day process and written about it,* I myself almost lost my position as head of medical services, ironically almost three years after the event. The powers that be tried to force me to warn against the process and advise people not to embark on it. This would have diametrically contradicted my view of science, so there was no question of my complying. It is to the credit of my superiors that they allowed me to retain my position despite protests from other colleagues. One aspect of this whole affair impressed me almost more than anything else: that in our seemingly so enlightened world of science, willingness to test and question basic concepts has if anything decreased but certainly not increased since the time of Galileo.

The phenomenon of receiving nourishment without food has fascinated me for decades. Even as a boy at grammar school I was passionately interested in reading accounts of yogis and saints. I have always been firmly convinced that those accounts speak the truth, and that we shall take a giant step forward in our

---

*Jasmuheen, 1998.

understanding of the world and in our level of scientific awareness if we recognize these phenomena. Reports about human abstinence from food and drink thrilled me as being possible harbingers of an expanded scientific and religious view of the world that might guide us away from the oppressive prison of today's materialism.

On a Saturday in November 1997 I discovered the book *Living on Light** by Ellen Greve alias Jasmuheen in a bookshop. I read it from cover to cover over the weekend and – thanks to a whole string of coincidences – found myself participating in a workshop conducted by Jasmuheen the very next weekend. Before I had even finished reading the book I knew that I would embark on the process. I needed direct contact with Jasmuheen in order to hear and sense whether her message seemed trustworthy, and also accounts by 'ordinary mortals' who had gone through the process and could thus reassure me that I would not be embarking on an irresponsible medical experiment. My conviction that it was basically possible to receive nourishment without food did not mean that it was advisable or without risk for average individuals leading average lives.

Despite insufficient preparation I found that my conversion to living without food or drink went astonishingly smoothly. From reports I had read I expected to feel increasingly weak during the early days. But then I began to realize that in my case this weakness was not going to happen. Instead I experienced an increasing sensation of levity and alertness during the day and a decrease in the amount of sleep I needed at night. Going through the process was probably the most intense experience of my adult life. The second and third weeks took an unexpected turn. Many old feelings and dreams which I had worked through in

---

* Jasmuheen, 1998.

therapy 25 years earlier, and believed finished and done with, resurfaced again. This took the form mainly of physical pain, feelings and cramps — chiefly in the abdominal region — and suchlike. Daily treatments by the healer Graziella Schmidt always took away the symptoms and returned me to a sense of wellbeing. Repeatedly I thought that all the old ballast of those feelings had been taken from me, only to find that a new wave swept over me again the following day. I gained an entirely new attitude to psychosomatic phenomena through experiencing how matters which appear to have been dealt with and which have been more or less banished from consciousness can still exist in one's 'cell memory' where they remain inaccessible to verbal therapies yet can be reached by the powers of a healer which we do not yet fully comprehend.

During the first seven days, when one also abstains from fluids, and because I needed less sleep, I usually danced intensively and joyously for up to two hours in the early morning between 4 and 6 a.m. The music, the movement and my increasing sense of physical levity often engendered an almost ecstatic state of overwhelming happiness. The combination of this with the resurfacing of old feelings led to constant ups and downs, sometimes agonizing, between the waves of psychological and physical pain from earlier sources and the repeated sensations of levity, happiness, gratitude and humility. Graziella's humour and my emotional levity meant that I have scarcely ever laughed as much as I did during those three weeks.

Does the process leading to 'living on light' have any social significance? At the present time hardly, at least not in the sense hoped for by Jasmuheen that ill-fed people in poor countries might be able to readjust the use of their inner energy and thus become less dependent on food. Perhaps this is something for the distant future, but for us today it remains theoretical.

At present the main concern is to expand scientific thinking or indeed the way we all think about the nature of our existence. The rapid transformation in awareness that we are now experiencing in society at large forms the background against which the phenomenon discussed in this book has its place. In this sense it can become one stone in the mosaic of the long path of humanity back to God, or back to a recognition of our fundamentally divine nature.

Preface

by Michael Werner

The idea of co-authoring a book on the subject of 'living on light' arose as a logical next step which followed quite quickly from work on an article for the weekly journal *Das Goetheanum*.* Our decision to go ahead was further strengthened by the positive and uncomplicated way in which we were able to collaborate, and above all by increasing calls and requests for more in-depth information.

The overall plan was clear to us from the start. It would be necessary not only to present an account of the theory in so far as it existed and could be coherently expressed, but above all to provide much practical information on the background and possibility of converting to a new way of receiving nourishment based on the experiences of those who had done it. I was greatly helped by what I had learned in connection with giving lectures on the subject of 'living on light', since I found that many people have an urgent need to ask questions which they have either been wrestling with for some time or which have arisen during the lecture itself; and if possible also to receive answers. Many understandable concerns have had to be or still are met with disappointing replies. There are so many questions which we cannot yet answer but which we do not want to dismiss with superficially intellectual rejoinders or theoretical put-downs. In such cases we prefer to admit to not knowing, or else we remain silent on the matter.

---

* Stockli, 2002.

In describing my practical experiences I have received much help from those I have been privileged to accompany on their journey through the 21-day process. They have enriched my own experience with their entirely individual and personal accounts, and I here take the opportunity to express my heartfelt gratitude to them. Approaching the phenomenon of 'living on light' must surely be only one of many endeavours to make full, or at least better, use of the possibilities which are given to all of us today or which we have allotted to ourselves. It is irrelevant in all this whether we adapt entirely to 'living on light' or not. The point is to experience, for example by following the 21-day process, the relative importance physical nourishment occupies in our lives.

Most of the people I know personally who have embarked on the 21-day process have sooner or later reverted to normal eating. In each case the reasons for this are entirely individual. Ingrained habit, social pressure, the pleasure of eating and so on can trigger the return to eating and drinking in the accustomed manner, as can a kind of lassitude that overtakes some by the end of the 21-day process. Some people are disappointed in themselves or in the process as such. This is not a problem as far as I can see, since the 21-day process as such is merely the first step towards 'living on light', and the distance covered by any one person is of course an individual matter. I do not know anyone who broke off in the middle of the process or who suffered any damage by seeing it through. Neither do I know anyone who regrets having made the effort. On the contrary, in every case the experience was felt to have been unique, beautiful, important and interesting.

My advice to those wanting to undergo the 21-day process is: Approach it with all the seriousness you can muster and with a willingness to take responsibility for applying your critical faculties to yourself; yet at the same time be relaxed and do not prejudge the outcome. Eating and drinking is not our main concern; what matters is what we experience and how we handle it. Our education and culture train us to look for either/or situations, and this is usually the wrong way to go about things, or even a hindrance. If the intention is to convert to 'living on light' it could be natural, safe and appropriate to approach this by eating and not eating in an alternating rhythm of first one, then the other. This would lead to greater freedom and awareness in the way one deals with matters of food and nutrition and make it possible to decide which way of handling these things fits one's own personal life situation at any given moment.

This book does not claim to have exhausted the subject of 'living on light', and much will in future no doubt have to be corrected, omitted, expanded or reformulated. Nevertheless, we hope that the considerations here will go some way towards fulfilling many enquirers' evident need for objective and reliable information. And of course there is no guarantee that during or after reading the book one will not end up with other as yet unanswered questions, perhaps even more than before.

PART ONE: EXPERIENCES

1

Who is Michael Werner?

by Thomas Stöckli

Michael Werner, born 1949 in Brunswick, Northern Germany, now lives in Switzerland, near Basle. With a PhD in chemistry, he has for the last 19 years been managing director of a pharmaceutical research institute at Arlesheim. He is married to a school teacher and has three teenage children. After working for many years in the chemical industry, also in South Africa, he taught chemistry and biology at a Waldorf (Steiner) school in Germany for three years.

Having taken virtually no solid food since January 2001,* he has also from time to time gone for longer periods completely without liquids, the longest span so far being ten days.

I have known him for five years and am now in regular contact with him. I know his family, his home and his colleagues at work; and over the whole of this period I have been observing him with growing interest, for the number of my questions has not decreased. The bewildering thing about him is that apart from having no need to eat, and practising this with total consistency, he is an 'entirely normal person' – indeed he refers to himself as 'Mr Ordinary'. As a scientist for whom life also holds a spiritual dimension, however, he feels it is important to share in bringing about the paradigm change which he feels is imminent. As he never ceases to point out, his concern is the imperative necessity to hold a question mark over our one-sided view of the world. And

---

* See also p. 52.

he endeavours to do this not by working out new theories but by presenting 'hard facts' and demonstrable physical phenomena.

The first article about Michael Werner and his form of 'living on light' appeared in September 2002,* but it had taken a long time for it to reach publication. The editorial team of the journal in question initially found it somewhat questionable and did not want to go ahead without having prior discussions and adding some kind of disclaimer. Since then, reactions to the article have been entirely positive, both from those in Werner's immediate environment and from complete strangers. He has received many letters and queries including some from a number of individuals who intended, on the basis of what they had read in the article, to 'convert' their eating habits by applying the '21-day process'. Some of their reports will be found in this book. The effect of that article is still ongoing, with the number of invitations to lecture increasing year on year. The dam appears to have burst, so that the subject which had been entirely taboo is becoming increasingly acceptable and up for discussion.

Meeting Michael Werner

My first meeting with Michael Werner was in 2001, shortly before Christmas. After a festive dinner at a teachers' training course – the table laden with a gorgeous selection of specialities from Africa, Russia and Switzerland – I had the opportunity to have a talk with him. I had heard from a friend that for almost a year he had not taken any food and also no longer had any need for it. Following my study of Nicholas von der Flüe I had accepted that there had been people – and even now there could be such – who could find nourishment other than by physical food. I had read Jasmuheen's book, and had heard there were, in

---

* Stöckli, 2002.

our time, people who were nourished by 'light', 'prana' or 'ether forces'. I felt somewhat antipathetic towards the book itself on account of its style and content. I found it to be a dangerous counsellor, with its esoteric potpourri and its '21-day process' describing how to abstain totally from food.

My friend, however, had confirmed to me the serious character of Michael Werner — for they were colleagues — and also of his many years of intensive involvement with serious spiritual work. So I had resolved to meet this person.

To take no food for a year and to work in a responsible position as quite a 'normal' and respected colleague, as well as being a family man and scientist, a chemist actually, sounded somewhat unbelievable!

To refute a materialistic world-view

I intended to research this matter seriously and furthermore to suggest that this case should be clinically examined. I was motivated by the following: If it is true that someone could live and be fit and healthy without eating or even drinking, then our conceptions as to what a human being needs to exist are quite practically refuted and this presents us with fundamental questions. Through this unusual phenomenon, perhaps deeper and wider ideas regarding human life in general could be developed.

When I interviewed Werner for the first time, he responded quite openly and spontaneously to my questions. Since 1 January 2001 he had no longer taken any solid food. He still joined in at mealtimes for social reasons, even cooking for his family at times, but since that time did not feel any hunger or thirst. He still drank coffee, various teas, fruit-juices and water, altogether taking between one half and a litre of liquid per day.

He said that he could also go without drinking and had done so for a whole week on three occasions. He was feeling much better than ever before. In the year of 'conversion' he had come to a crisis point physically: a fractured leg, a spine operation and bladder and kidney problems – giving him the feeling that his body, at 51 years of age, was disintegrating. And yet now he was feeling in tip-top condition physically, emotionally, mentally and also with regard to his memory and ability to concentrate. He needed noticeably less sleep, engaged in sports and did his work with enjoyment and engagement.

At our second meeting, at his home on a cool day in May, we sat outside in his garden. I felt chilled by the cool breeze whereas he was in good form, full of activity, using his short midday break for a further talk with me and with his wife before returning on foot, as usual, to his place of work. At the age of 52 he certainly did not give the impression of a starving person, with his sun-tanned complexion and determined gait.

The whole story still seemed so incomprehensible, and it was important to me to get to know his personal environment in order to arrive at a more comprehensive picture. His wife willingly agreed to a meeting and told me that naturally she had followed everything from close quarters. She spoke of how her husband had fared since the 'conversion'. Strangely, she was confident that it would work out well, but in the beginning she had had great doubts as to whether their family life would change radically. Her husband was formerly very fond of food and they had often cooked together for the family. At first it had been a strange thing for the three children to have their father sitting at the table without a plate. But now everything was running without any problems, their private and family life much as it was before. She did mention that neighbours and acquaintances who knew of this change in her husband could not cope with the subject – one simply didn't speak about it…

'Living on light' – a free decision and an offer by the spiritual world

In our very first conversation Werner told me how he had met with the idea of undergoing this 'conversion':

'I had heard of this possibility from a good acquaintance. I then read Jasmuheen's book *Living on Light*, but was not particularly impressed by it. Yet, because of this person I was acquainted with, I recognized that somehow such a phenomenon was a reality – and this reality had something to do with myself. This was early in the summer of 2000. After some months of pondering and examining myself, I decided to undertake the so-called "21-day process". To be frank, curiosity was also part of my motivation. Does it work? And if so – how? I decided to follow the practical advice given in the book. I never had a bad feeling about it. I also knew I would be able to call it off at any time. I was utterly free, it was my own decision, and that was of central importance to me.'

In answer to my question as to how his experience differed from fasting, he replied: 'This is something totally different! With fasting the body mobilizes reserves of substances and forces; you cannot fast for an unlimited time, neither can you go without drinking. But this process I was undertaking was and remains a mental-spiritual phenomenon and requires a special inner tuning. There is actually only one condition: that I can open myself to the thought that I can be nourished by light, by the *etheric*, by *prana* or whatever it may be called. This is the bridge that is needed. Then it will happen. I experienced it as an offer by the spiritual world.

'In the first seven days I did not drink even a drop of liquid.

The general view is that you cannot live for more than five days without liquid. But you experience in your own body that this is wrong! Suddenly, you experience that these generally held views do not tally with reality. If someone dies of thirst or hunger, it is because of his or her environment. There is the conviction that without drinking and eating one has to die. This has been the case hitherto, but for the last 15–20 years we have been living in another field of energy with new possibilities. Of course, history shows that there have been exceptional personalities, such as Nicholas von der Flüe or Therese of Konnersreuth – also yogis – who could do this, but for quite normal people, such as myself, this was beyond reach. This is now a new and apparently special dispensation from the spiritual world.'

I could somehow imagine that this was possible – Nicholas von der Flüe's total renunciation of food had not overturned my view of the world. But I asked myself: What good will this serve? Eating is not only enjoyable, but is also a social activity, closely uniting us with the earth. Werner agreed that this actual point poses the greatest problem. Yet, for him it was not just a question of eating and drinking. It was his evident experience that the generally accepted view of a material-physical world is incorrect:

'The materialistic world-view can be refuted theoretically, but today this is no longer sufficient. It requires practical, quite concrete proof. Yet all of a sudden my close acquaintances also have a problem with me!' Even some scientists associated with the work of the Austrian-born 'spiritual scientist' Rudolf Steiner* – with which Michael Werner is connected – are not more open.

---

* 1861–1924. Rudolf Steiner founded the art and science of anthroposophy, a discipline that incorporates methods of personal development and philosophical and spiritual investigation, as well as fresh approaches to practical activities in fields such as medicine, agriculture, education, architecture, and so on. See also Appendix.

In other words, everyone reacts individually. He is experiencing the whole scale of responses: from interest and openness right through to denial and defensiveness. Nevertheless, he was greatly astonished that hardly anyone had shown any *serious* interest in this phenomenon. 'Somehow I have the feeling: it is simply too much for most people. They repress it; for every scientist it causes anxiety that they will have to revise their world-view.'

I sensed Werner's disappointment. Yet he could also appreciate those people who meet the phenomenon with an open mind. I felt I was one such person. A modern spiritual world view presents ways of thinking that allow the unusual to be admitted in principle and all phenomena to be taken seriously. Only after a careful assessment should a judgement be made. And yet I found that Jasmuheen's book still brought up a number of problems for me. For this reason I probed again: 'What is your position with regard to some of the highly pro-blematical aspects of the so-called "New Age?"' He replied: 'I cannot say anything regarding the person of Jasmuheen. I know too little about her. Concerning her book, readers have to use their own discrimination in judging it. The centre of the book – some thirty pages describing the "conversion" – is not written by Jasmuheen but by Charmaine Harley and is, in my opinion, fine. One can easily have questions about the rest of the book. I can only repeat that personally I have not experienced the pro-cess of "conversion" as life-threatening. I always knew that I could stop at any time. After all, every dogmatic and radical attitude can present a danger to life.'

Matter as 'condensed light'

For me there were still points of conflict. I continued to question Werner's spiritual path, and whether, since his 'conversion', he had had any specific spiritual experiences. 'For the last 25 years I have lived intensively with anthroposophy and have worked out my own spiritual path of inner exercises. I was able to deepen my meditation and my spiritual endeavours. My deeper connection with the spiritual world did not happen automatically by renouncing physical food, but because I strive for it. One does not slip effortlessly into the spiritual. I could never be party to such a path. I am left entirely free. Neither is there any organization posing any expectations or obligations on me. I myself know of no other person practising this, except the acquaintance I have mentioned.'

I kept on probing: As a scientist, how could he explain to himself the phenomenon of 'living on light'? Werner's answer was: 'I have read everything by Rudolf Steiner concerning the process of nutrition and have found nothing that I have experienced as problematic with regard to this phenomenon, but neither have I found any direct explanation. The closest bridge I found was in a lecture in which Steiner said that matter is "condensed light".* Matter, therefore, is light and there are different ways to turn light into matter. The concept "light" would not apply in too narrow a sense. It is the whole "etheric" [life] environment, which we can "inhale" with our whole sensory organization, as Steiner repeatedly explained. This could be called "living on light". After eating and drinking, our body breaks down the material aspect completely and it is then partly restructured and enlivened anew in order to build us up and maintain us. This helps the body to maintain its structural principles. "Living on light" would in some senses be a simplification of this process, in that the body does not require solid matter but receives its building substances and structuring

---

* R. Steiner, 1995 (see lecture of 27 May 1910).

forces directly from other sources. I can only say that through this phenomenon I have found an entirely new relationship to my body and to earthly substances. I experience it in a very inward way, yet without turning away from matter and the earth. Connected with this, however, is also an act of consciousness in that, by devotion and turning towards physical substances around me, I cultivate a conscious relationship. Otherwise, it might perhaps go astray and become a lower egotism. Even when we talk about "living on light" we are not concerned with the effects of physical light. Light, as such, is in any case invisible. What matters is the whole energy-environment, which we may call "ether-forces".'

To become an 'icebreaker' – to overcome scepticism

Scepticism, and usually also disbelief of this extraordinary phenomenon, can surely only be cleared away by strict scientific testing.* I therefore asked Werner how he would respond to a scientific project in which he would be isolated for 3–4 weeks, observed minutely and medically tested. Werner stressed that he would willingly cooperate fully with such an experiment. He added that physiological tests had already been done on him. A thorough examination at a university clinic had produced medical results that his blood plasma, as well as its chemical composition, his urine and basic metabolism and respiratory system revealed no exceptional data – there were no deviations from accepted normal standards. All of this is, of course, not yet convincing to the sceptics – could he be eating secretly? Only a scientifically designed and monitored experiment could establish the phenomenon as concrete fact. For Werner this would mean a positive challenge to

---

* See more about this on pages 130–158 and 215–219.

science 'in the classical sense'. Science has always made progress through such challenges. People are needed in our scientific establishments who can muster the courage to become 'icebreakers'.

2

Michael Werner's lectures on receiving nourishment from light

by Thomas Stöckli

Michael Werner's concerns and ideas are best expressed in his lectures. Speaking to an audience challenges him to give clear explanations and descriptions of what he thinks and has experienced, and his open replies to critical questions from his audience provide ample food for reflection even if they fail to convince the sceptics. As an example we here include the record of a lecture 'Food from Light – Questioning the Materialistic View of the World, Lecture and Conversation with Dr Michael Werner, Chemist, Dornach, Switzerland' given in Stuttgart, Germany, in May 2004 to an audience of about 400. The organizer, Ulrich Morgenthaler, had the following to say about the wider aspects and mood of that lecture:

I had seen a photo of him and we had exchanged a few e-mails. On meeting him face to face I found him more reserved than I had expected. He observed his surroundings including myself with interest tinged with a kind of inner objectivity as though looking in from the distant location of his own quietness. This was enhanced by a stance that made him appear to be leaning backwards slightly. He did not come across as someone with a message to impart but more like an individual who is himself curious to discover where he is going, alert to whom and whatever he might meet. He smiled slightly as though enjoying an adventure.

I had invited him to supper and asked him to arrive in Stuttgart two hours before the lecture to give us time to get to know each other. It was only in the middle of preparing the hall that I realized my faux pas: I've invited him to a meal, but he doesn't eat anything! How embarrassing! But Michael Werner had accepted the invitation. While I ate he sat beside me, taking pleasure at my enjoyment of the tasty food. He himself had ordered an espresso: 'Because this is what I like!' he said. We discussed the evening. He would make the lecture short because he was more interested in entering into conversation with people and hearing their questions about 'living on light'.

Five hundred people came. In spite of an overflow facility and much improvisation in the corridors we had to turn away over 100. Disappointed faces. Why had so many turned up? The subject of obtaining nourishment from light is not as new as all that. For years there have been people living without solid or liquid food, including some who have spoken in public about it. There are books. There are internet sites. Nonetheless it appears to be an entirely new and challenging theme for many people.

From the start everyone listened intently, because he was speaking from experience. 'Is it possible to live without eating or drinking? Yes.' This said it all, right at the beginning, and it was convincing. Only someone who has experienced it and is experiencing it could sound so convincing. Michael Werner's quiet voice gave a direct sense of what he has done and the path he has trodden. In a way, no further explanations were necessary. He caught the attention of his audience who were fully alert in their expectant enjoyment at perhaps discovering something new in hitherto dark corners of the mind. This overall impression put its stamp on the lecture for me, but there were surely also some who were sceptical about what the speaker had to say.

The subject concerns everyone, for what Werner has experienced is not an individual matter. If it were, he said, he would not speak about it. It was precisely because his opening statement was generally valid and applied to anyone that he did speak about 'living on light'. Such sentences hit home and while people listened they began to question their own deeply-rooted attitudes to life. And then he turned to his chief motivation: He hoped there would be questions from those present, and he reckoned they would take yet more questions home with them. It was not a matter of eating and drinking, or that there were others who also stopped eating and drinking. What he wanted was for his audience to begin thinking about eating and drinking in a different way. This process of awareness was the most important thing for him.

Michael Werner knows quite well that the subject of 'living on light' is passed on from person to person. Just as he was now speaking about it to others, so had his attention initially been drawn to it by someone else. So he felt it to be important to speak about his own reaction. The subject had moved him personally, and he had known: 'One day, I shall do that!' And he also stressed what finally gave rise to his embarking on 'living on light': a serious illness. He encouraged people to observe and listen in to their own lives.

But there was one basic requirement: one must believe in the possibility of receiving nourishment from light or, even better, one must be open to the idea. That is when things become objectively exciting, for in his opinion the ability to 'live on light' was not the same in days gone by as it is today. The question remained in the air: what was this about a connection between the need to be convinced as to the possibility of 'living on light' and a change in the situation of the time? If the possibility of 'living on light' depends on one's own conscious attitude, would it not be necessary for consciousness to have the character of light and for light to have consciousness or some kinship with the content of thoughts? And if it was not possible to live on light in the past in the way it is possible today, has light changed, or the character of human consciousness, or the possibility for the human being to shape his own consciousness? And who or what brings about such changes?

This was not a lecture. It was a personal account. And the tension and intensity came about because such questions were raised but not put into words or talked about.

After a good hour he brought his account to an end. Intently and expectantly he waited for questions from the floor. He had left many questions open and also pointed out that there would be many he couldn't answer. But he hoped that questions would set a process in motion through which he, too, would find new perspectives opening up. He himself wanted to go into the matter more deeply, to investigate and discover new things, and he hoped those present would help. One element in all this is surely that as a practising chemist Michael Werner is himself a scientist and therefore also a researcher. So he is motivated from the start to be profoundly interested in discovering and understanding new things. Hence we can also understand how, as an anthroposophist*, he came to get involved in something that did not originate in anthroposophy but came from quite a different esoteric source.

The discussion which lasted almost an hour and a half generated an atmosphere full of shared activity and attentiveness. In comparing this with other talks one is tempted to ask how it was possible for so many intensive and for the most part pertinent and important questions to come about. How much was due to the sensational nature of the theme, and how much to the way the subject matter was presented? Part of the lively interest of course came from the subject matter as such. But I'm sure the main reason for it stemmed from Werner himself. By leaving aside detailed explanations and not exploring every

---

* Somebody who follows the path of anthroposophy, see footnote on p. 20.

aspect to the bitter end, by restricting his report to a concise description of what he himself had been through and of his own inner and outer experiences of the phenomena, he had created a space in which his audience could become aware of their own questions.

Another aspect was also the way he conducted himself. If he had no answer to a question he simply said: 'I don't know.' And if he described a fact for which he had no explanation, again he just said: 'Well, that's how it is.' There was a lightness in the way he came across that might have given rise to an impression almost of heedlessness but which also helped people to open up in a carefree way to the adventure of 'living on light'. Coupled with his dry humour including his ability to poke fun at himself, all this contributed to a empathetic, open-minded atmosphere that enabled listeners to approach him openly and directly with their own questions and comments.

The event ended officially after three hours. But even then people didn't want to go straight home. Many crowded round the speaker to continue talking about various aspects of his subject. Michael Werner evidently meets with this high degree of interest wherever he talks publicly about his experiences. This subject is a true phenomenon of our time, a sign of the transformation and expansion of consciousness that is coming about among us human beings.

Other lectures by Werner have also left a deep impression on people. For example one he gave in Solothurn in May 2003 ended with a 76-year-old local gentleman declaring that he, too, had followed the 21-day process, since when he had not eaten for the past nine months; his description was delightfully humorous and refreshing. Again, that evening of lecturing was special. Here was someone speaking not of wise spiritual matters he had read about but of personal experiences, a 'witness to spiritual events' talking in well-grounded, objective tones. The modest and sober style of the two speakers created a concentrated mood that was both full of tension and relaxed, humorous and refreshing. And nothing at all gave the impression of people wanting to put across a message or beat the drum of propaganda.

Sometimes, as we have said, Michael Werner replies to a question from the audience by saying: 'I don't know.' And then he proceeds to feel his way towards a possible answer. Here we see the honest scientist who does not make sensational, wild claims but modestly allows the phenomena to speak for themselves without coming to premature conclusions. He has a lively interest in serious research into the phenomenon. He is both a practitioner and a theoretician, truly a practical researcher.

On hearing about the phenomenon of 'living on light' for the first time, many people are astonished and impressed at first but then also quickly tend to poke fun at the whole thing. But the ridicule soon falls silent when they have the opportunity to meet someone who actually does obtain nourishment from light, someone who is neither terribly thin nor ill, neither off with the fairies nor hypersensitive, but who on the contrary is full of vitality, is healthy and modest, in short a normal individual in the best sense of the words.

The lecture

by Michael Werner

'Yes', is the only answer I can give to the question 'Is it possible to live without eating?' Let me explain in a bit more detail, since this is rather an unusual question and also an unusual answer. I don't intend to give the ordinary kind of lecture but rather a report many parts of which will be quite personal. This has advantages and disadvantages. One advantage is that what is said gains a degree of immediacy: here's someone speaking from experience. A disadvantage is that being very personal it may be rather one-sided. However, what I want to tell you about is not in the least individual. I shall be telling you personal things which I am quite sure also apply to others.

I shall tell you what I have done, what happened when I did it, and how the original idea came to me. I shall then attempt to give a few explanations. For example it is possible to find some leads in anthroposophy that can help us gain an understanding of the phenomenon of 'living on light'. Afterwards we can talk about all this, and the questions that have occurred to you or that you perhaps brought here with you. I'm sure you came here with some questions and I hope that you will go home with yet more.

There is one point that should be clear from the start: I am not at all concerned about whether you eat and drink or whether you now intend to cease eating and drinking. This is not what I am concerned with. I'm not concerned with eating and drinking since in itself this is not very interesting but merely a means to an end. To me what is important is that you might begin to think about these things in a different way. If this were to happen it would be great. This brings us to the subtitle of today's lecture, 'Questioning the Materialistic View of the World', but we'll come to that later.

How it came about

So the answer to the question 'Can we live without eating and drinking?' is 'Yes, we can.' I have done it myself and am still doing it. So now let me try to describe it in more detail.

I'm a perfectly normal person. If I were an exception there would surely be no point in telling my story. I had been engaged with spiritual matters for a long time and had gained a certain amount of experience in the field. But then all of a sudden I quite unexpectedly found myself confronted with the phenomenon of 'living on light'. This may have been what people call a coincidence, or perhaps it was providence. An old acquaintance of my wife came to visit us, a woman I too had known for many years. We immediately noticed that she had grown very thin, almost haggard. And here she was, paying us a visit but — not eating anything. When we asked what was the matter and did she have a problem she simply said she was not eating any longer. Then she told us she had followed a special programme, changed her way of life and now 'lived on light'. I was immediately very taken by this. Of course we talked about it and she gave me a detailed account of what she had done and why. As we talked I immediately realized: One day I shall do this too.

Being a scientist, a chemist, I was spontaneously attracted to the idea. I never had any real problems and I also never thought: That's impossible. I had heard of Nicholas von der Flüe and Therese of Konnersreuth and had also read the relevant description of her in Yogananda's *Autobiography of a Yogi*. But I had always assumed that these were exceptional people who could live without taking any nourishment because of their destiny, or by the grace of God as a revelation of certain phenomena, or through a quirk of nature. That it might be possible for any 'Mr Ordinary' was entirely new to me. But now here I was, faced with this very possibility.

This happened four years ago at a time when I was quite unwell. I was very overweight, had high blood pressure and all kinds of symptoms that I won't go into here. This was another good reason for considering such an experiment. Nine months passed while I thought about it. I also developed even more complaints. So finally I said to myself: This is it; I'm going to do it. So I changed my way of receiving nourishment and since then I no longer live on food and drink. But neither do you, my friends. Only you don't realize it. In the final analysis we all more or less 'live on light'. Usually this takes a detour via the plants which assimilate light and convert it into sugar and other substances, thus binding forces. Actually, life is impossible without light, and this is a life force which we can absorb directly. To call this 'living on light' is just one of many possible labels. We can just as truthfully speak of the etheric, or *prana*, or *chi*, or cosmic energy. These are all one and the same thing. It is a natural, divine energy that is present everywhere in abundance.

How does 'it' work?

How can something like this be done? It's quite simple. You just have to get on with it, you have to permit it to happen, and then it functions almost of its own accord. There is, however, one important precondition, and that is that you must believe that it is possible to 'live on light'. Or to put it in another, perhaps better, way: You have to open yourself to it, you have to trust it. This is perhaps most important and indeed decisive. You see, when I converted to doing it I'm not so sure that I actually believed in it. But what I did was expect it with a fundamentally open mind.

This is what is possible nowadays, whereas in former times it was probably not so much a matter of course. I know a number of people who have undertaken the process, and I'm sure there are very many more. But those I know are enough for me to be sure that it really does work.

The 21-day process

The process of converting to 'living on light' has been described in detail by Jasmuheen in her eponymous book. I am not too keen on the book itself, but the part on the actual process of conversion is well-written and clear; the instructions can be followed almost like following a recipe in a cookbook. I recommend anyone who wants to try to convert to read that text and mark it well. (See chapter 3 'On the 21-day process'.)

It takes three weeks, hence the designation '21-day process'. This is surely not arbitrary, for 3 times 7 covers rhythms we have within us. I began to follow the process quite suddenly at the beginning of 2001. Of course I did prepare myself, especially mentally. But then I went straight into it. I celebrated New Year's Eve with my family and still remember eating potato salad and cake and drinking coffee. And then, on the stroke of midnight, that was it!

I shall describe the actual conversion process in more detail to show you that it doesn't just drop from the skies. You do have to do it yourself, you have to open yourself to it. The absolute rule for the first week is: 'Eat nothing and drink nothing!' And that really does mean not a crumb and not a drop. Any physician will tell you that it's impossible. You can fast for 40 or even 50 days, but to drink nothing for seven is impossible. In general it is considered that a human being can survive for five days without drinking. For example, in the days when Christians set out on their voyages of discovery from Europe, the sailors used to say with reference to accidents at sea: For three days we are thirsty, on the fourth we go crazy, and on the fifth we die. Why is this? And why do thousands of people starve to death every day? It is simply that they are convinced they will starve if they have nothing to eat.

It is perfectly possible to live for seven days without drinking. But it is pretty radical. You lose a lot of weight and you get dehydrated. And there are a number of symptoms, some more and some less unpleasant, which occur and which you should definitely know about beforehand.

My experiences during the 21-day process

Very sensibly one is urgently advised for the whole of the conversion period to withdraw entirely from everyday life and avoid any kind of daily stress; so take a holiday. One is naturally very weak and needs rest, but it is nevertheless a most beautiful and special experience.

At the beginning it feels rather like the kind of fast that you undertake as a cure at a spa. You soon get a headache because your body is beginning to detoxify. This detoxification also often causes the tongue to be coated and swollen. It feels furry and you have a bad taste in the mouth just as you usually do when fasting.

A change takes place after three or four days. In my case I woke up on the fourth day and immediately realized: this is no longer just fasting. And I had the definite feeling: Now everything is alright. The rule in the second week is: 'Eat nothing, but do drink.' So again you take not a crumb of solid food, but you drink diluted juice (25 per cent diluted fruit juice), as much as you like. The first sip is like a ceremony, a celebration, and feels absolutely wonderful. The main purpose of this drinking is to detoxify the body so that it can adapt to the new way of receiving nourishment. In the third week you still do not eat, but your fruit juices need less diluting (about 40 per cent). Orange juice is best. Drinking in the second week stabilizes the new situation. You notice this quite clearly; you feel stronger and gain a little weight. At the end of the 21 days the process is complete. You can then do exactly what you like. You might start eating again, or just continue drinking, or not even that. Just as you wish, and whatever seems meaningful and suitable for your own situation and personal needs.

Throughout the process it is important to be aware that you are entirely free to decide what you want to do. You can break off at any stage, but I can report that I know of no one who has done this. But being aware that it is up to you puts your mind at rest and gives you a feeling of confidence. I myself began the process with certain provisos and had decided simply to stop if anything appeared abnormal or if something untoward occurred. But this was not the case.

After the 21-day process

Having finished the 21 days I then stopped drinking again, just to see what would happen. I started to lose more weight, and so started drinking again. Over the three weeks I had anyway lost a great deal of weight, about 15 kg, and looked like a shrivelled-up tortoise. So I began drinking again and thus stabilized my weight and my appearance with the help of fruit juices. Since then I drink something at every mealtime, sometimes water, sometimes tea or herb tea, sometimes coffee depending on the situation and what I fancy. From the beginning I decided never to miss a meal or exclude myself from mealtimes. I always take an active part in every meal; in addition to nourishing the body, eating also has an important social element. You sit together, in a manner of speaking you eat from one bowl, the children come home from school and need to offload their stress and worries; you share experiences and exchange ideas.

I have observed that most people who undertake the 21-day process go back to eating and drinking again at some point. Social pressure, enjoying food, or habit are the main reasons; but there are others too. The social element is the strongest, and I myself still experience this frequently, although on the whole I now know what to expect in most situations and have become relatively thick-skinned in this respect. What I mean to say is that it is not entirely easy to handle social situations that arise in connection with 'living on light'. But I must also stress once more that people should feel free to do exactly as they wish. Starting to eat again is not a problem, not even physiologically. Every individual must make up his or her own mind and find out what is most comfortable.

Good friends, and also my mother, frequently ask: 'When are you going to start eating again?' The only answer I can give is: 'I don't know.' At the moment, after over three years without food, I feel so well, in fact better than ever, that I'd be a fool to start eating again. So long as I feel well I shall not eat. Perhaps I shall begin again one day, but I have no fixed idea about this.

Physiological and medical facts

I am no specialist in matters of physiology, but as time has gone on a number of things have become clear to me. On the other hand many questions remain unanswered, and new ones have arisen as well.

My personal experience is as follows: I began 'living on light' just after turning 51. Healthwise I was in a difficult situation and this was one of the reasons that seriously motivated me to make the change, which from that point of view has been of great benefit to me. I have since had no need to consult the doctor on any chronic physical matters. Of course this doesn't mean that 'living on light' is a panacea, but it is certainly a very good way of keeping more healthy than one would otherwise be. In my case, I got rid of my surplus weight and my weight has since remained stable at a good low level depending on how much I drink or exercise. Please believe me: I really do feel very well. My body is fit, and I have even noticed that injuries heal well and more quickly than before. Former problems, for example high blood pressure which was surely linked to being overweight, have returned to normal. All in all I feel perfectly robust.

Since I began I have been examined medically several times and am always relieved to hear that everything is normal, whether in blood or urine, which only goes to confirm what I feel.

Beyond the physiological

Obtaining one's nourishment in this way of course also involves other important and more profound aspects that go beyond the physical. Many and very varied motivations surely lie behind embarking on such a process, and in my case my physical health was not actually the central factor in my decision. Inwardly I was more interested or even fascinated in simply trying it out. And a considerable part in this was played by the possibility of discovering new and unfamiliar psychological and mental capacities. This expectation immediately proved valid in a good way. I feel much more stable emotionally and am mentally very much more alert and lively. I can concentrate much better; I need considerably less sleep and have plenty of vitality to get me through the day; and I simply feel very well.

Of course this way of obtaining nourishment doesn't work

miracles. I haven't become clairvoyant and I can't walk on water; but that's not what I'm after. I am, however, deeply convinced that anyone with ambitions of personal achievement in this sense would probably find 'living on light' a good and healthy basis on which to work towards reaching such goals. It can also provide an additional support in the healing of all kinds of illnesses even if the malady in question also necessitates undergoing certain healing processes as well. What I am trying to say is that 'living on light' is not a process that promises certain specific results.

How I experienced receiving nourishment through light

What happens when you obtain your nourishment in this way? How do you experience and perceive it? After the 21-day process, or indeed even during the first week, it was unequivocally clear to me that in some way or other I was receiving nourishment. I was being nourished in the sense that I felt: there is a force, a source, a living stream, some kind of life force that can be clearly sensed. This was not yet present in the first few days, but it suddenly manifested after about four, and it remains with me to this day. This is different from the ordinary process of being nourished. If you eat and drink in the normal way there is a rhythm of eating, digesting and then excreting. This is not the case when you live on light; or at least I have not noticed it. It is also not necessary to do anything in particular in order to be fed by this force.

In other words, being nourished by light is a continuous process and it runs of its own accord. In mentally accompanying this process I personally had my own individual meditations which I value, which I practise regularly and which I cultivated more intensively during the period of converting to a new way of receiving nourishment. But this is definitely not a precondition either for carrying out the process or for receiving nourishment in this way. One feels rather like a fish in water; it is permanently wet and can do whatever it fancies. This is what receiving nourishment from light feels like.

Naturally I also experience phases during everyday life when I feel exhausted. And when I get tired, usually around midnight, I have neither the inclination nor the strength to stay awake. However, I sleep relatively little, but nearly always deeply, and feel well rested when I wake up; and this is sufficient for the new day.

So 'living on light' is not the usual way of getting fed, which entails having to do something about it. It simply happens, like an unexpected gift, a benison.

Life energy

When you receive your nourishment from light, an energy or a force, or whatever you like to call it, flows into you; it is simply present when you need it. How much comes in depends on how much you use; this is like a law of nature. I do sport, for example, yet my condition is good, certainly much better than it used to be.

When I say I 'live on light' people often get the wrong end of the stick. They ask: 'Do you go out in the midday sun? Do you sunbathe while everyone else is having lunch?' Of course I don't, and it's also entirely unnecessary. To understand what I mean by 'light' in this context we need to define the concept more precisely. Normally when we talk of 'light' we visualize lightness and darkness and the variety of colours. This is inexact and is not light itself but the effect light has. Lightness and darkness and the various colours are not light but merely the effects of light. Light as such is invisible. It is everywhere, but we can only see its effects, for example when parts of it are reflected by material objects, causing colours to arise. Light also exists underneath the surface of the earth, so I'm sure it would also be possible to 'live on light' down there in the dark, at least for some time. So the term 'living on light' is actually misleading.

It is quite simply a ubiquitous energy that is everywhere present, and one of the ways in which it reveals itself is in light. Light forms the boundary between the material and the immaterial. It also has those delicately contrasting qualities arising from its wave nature on the one hand and its particle nature on the other, its wave-particle duality. It functions at the boundary between the material and the spiritual, which is why 'living on light' does after all remain the best way of describing it. But there is more to it than 'light' and 'nourishment', so it can also be called by the name of Christ, or Allah, or Krishna, or many others.

Getting to grips with understanding 'living on light'
It is difficult to explain the phenomenon and even more difficult to understand it. The idea of an energy that we take in from the air or the light is just about conceivable. But understanding how it relates to substance, matter, is considerably more difficult.

Normally one assumes that in everyday life energy and matter are incompatible and independent of one another, although since the discoveries and calculations of Albert Einstein every physicist knows that energy and matter are actually one and the same thing. We are accustomed to matter remaining stable and not being transformed into energy, and vice versa. But when it does happen, for example in the case of radioactive decay, it normally takes a very long time, while when it occurs suddenly, as in nuclear fission in a nuclear bomb, it takes place with uncontrollable, monstrous force. Huge amounts of energy are released, which is actually not so very surprising and is perfectly comprehensible to physicists.

If you eat nothing and drink only small amounts without any change in body weight, this appears to make no sense. A human being exhales approximately half a litre of water every day and loses a further half litre through the skin in order to maintain a constant temperature. So you'd think it would be necessary to drink at least a litre of water a day. And if you don't, while nevertheless maintaining a constant body weight, it doesn't add up. And if your hair and nails continue to grow, and your skin to flake and lose minerals through perspiration you can't help asking: 'Where does it all come from?' That is the decisive question: Where does it come from?

Rudolf Steiner's views on nourishment

I have been studying Rudolf Steiner's anthroposophy* for many years and have discovered bridges in his work that lead to a possible understanding of the phenomenon. In our under-standing of the world and life there is scarcely anything on which his vast work does not touch in some way. Although he never spoke directly about 'living on light' there are a number of indications that can take us further.

He said of matter, of substances, that all substances and all matter are, ultimately, 'condensed, compressed light'. They are solidified processes. We all know from experience that fluid, moving water can take on the form of steam which is extremely volatile and finely dispersed, and that a drop in temperature can turn it into ice, which is solid and immovable. This is an analogy that can be applied to Steiner's view that all matter is condensed, compressed light. As a starting point for understanding how light can provide nourishment this is a good beginning.

Steiner spoke a good deal about nourishment and food in a

---

* See Appendix.

number of lectures discussing what human beings need: proteins, fats, carbohydrates and minerals. On water, however, he strangely enough said very little. Yet in my opinion water is the most important. There is an interesting lecture in which Steiner used the potato as an example of how nourishment functions. He concluded his deliberations by describing how we only eat so that the exertion of digesting can stimulate the body to take in something from the etheric sphere, that is from the environment, from the general life forces around us which can then be transformed into the substances that maintain and build up our body. So we eat, for example, a potato. We chew it and digest it. This then stimulates us to absorb life forces from our etheric environment and condense them into substances. In other words, our body gains structure and substance by taking in light, or light forces, and condensing them. (See also p. 165.)

Questions from the floor

Basic questions

Question: You said just now that this method of receiving nourishment was in general not possible in former times. What was different then, and when did things change?

I am sure that living on light was only possible in exceptional cases in the past. I mentioned Nicholas von der Flüe and Therese of Konnersreuth as examples. Today, however, it is universally possible. It's a new phenomenon which as far as I am aware became known quite suddenly in Australia through channelling towards the end of the 1980s. Since then it has been practised and talked about. I do believe that prior to that it was not generally attainable; and I mean 'attainable', since it was of course known about earlier. My feeling is that with the world in such a parlous state at present, this possibility was created, or indeed had to be created as an aid to those who want to work at increasing their awareness. It provokes people to shake off their materialistic view of the world, whether through experiencing the phenomenon of 'living on light' themselves or through seeing it convincingly practised by others. And I am sure that this is a good thing.

Question: How has the situation changed? How did this new possibility come about?

It's quite simple. This is a gift from the spiritual world to us human beings. It is quite simply a new possibility. But it is also an experiment in which no one knows whether the goal of helping as many people as possible to gain new insights will in the end be reached. It's like the sun rising slowly in the morning and then gradually flooding the darkness with more and more light. After a while you can tell whether the mist and clouds are receding to leave the day warm and bright. It depends on many factors, so the end result cannot always be predicted.

Question: In Jasmuheen's book Living on Light *a great variety of origins is given with reference to the process. As helpers she mentions well-known and less well-known masters together with angelic beings from eastern and western esoteric traditions. What is your own attitude to this? And can you also see any Christian basis in it?*

As far as I know the path for humanity at large which is provided by the 21-day process is relatively new. I can only speculate about its origins and the reasons why it should appear just now. I imagine that receiving nourishment from light was not actually part of the plan for the straightforward onward development of humanity at the present time. The possibility has appeared suddenly and could not necessarily have been foreseen. It is evident that a critical situation has come about in the evolution of the earth. The spiritual world, I mean the good and positive spiritual beings and leaders of humanity, are watching planet earth and humanity with anxiety and despair because they see that the great majority of human beings are unable to break out of a materialism that is destructive and also no longer suitable for our time. In this sense, the phenomenon of 'living on light' is surely only one of many ways of helping to bring about an improvement in the situation.

Question: You have stated very emphatically that the process you have been describing is not a matter that concerns you alone. Is it really something anyone could do?
Yes, indeed. We all have the possibility of opening ourselves to receiving nourishment from light. But the decision to do this is of course an entirely personal matter. One must decide for oneself whether it is worthwhile, meaningful and necessary to follow this path. There is one precondition, however. If you want to convert your way of receiving nourishment you must have confidence and believe in the helping and nourishing forces that come from the spiritual world. So if anyone wants to try out 'living on light' with a positive and open mind, it will work. But you do of course really have to want it.

I know very well from personal experience of these things that many people have great difficulty in being unprejudiced, open and positive with regard to the phenomenon of 'living on light'. So in the final analysis there are not very many who are doing it or will do it.

Question: How many fellow contenders do you have? How many people are there who are 'living on light'?
I don't think anyone really knows, but I assume there may be a few thousand. The method has been known for several years, and people talk and write about it. Perhaps there are only a few hundred. I don't know. Personally I am acquainted with between twenty and thirty. But this is a completely arbitrary number and sample. What is more, presumably no one knows how many people there are who have come to be nourished by cosmic forces, by light or by prana through other means, like yogis who practise ascetic abstinence.

There is no clearly-defined or structured organization and no obvious collaboration. Of course you can glean some information through the internet, but this is very uncoordinated and I find it rather frustrating. Nevertheless it is a known 'movement' that has been spreading noticeably in recent years.

Question: I could imagine that a good many young people might become fascinated by the possibility of 'living on light'. Do you think there should be a warning about the problems?

I have already given a good many lectures on this subject, and there have always been some young people among the audience. Reactions have always been very positive, regardless of age. However, I can count on two hands the number of individuals who have been inspired by my talks actually to embark on the process. There has not been and there will not be a mass 'living on light' movement. The necessary step is too great, so that in the end only very few will cross this bridge. The practice actually generates its own protection against unthinking abuse. People who shouldn't do it don't even try. Actually this applies to many things in life, although it is always possible for individual cases to prove the exception or be dogged by an unfortunate conglomeration of circumstances.

Question: Thousands of helpless children starve to death every day. Could children carry out the 'living on light' process?

This would surely depend on the children and those who accompany them through the process, but in principle I think it would be possible. Once you accept the possibility that people today can be nourished by light, this can't be a matter of age. It's either possible or not possible. Whether children have the awareness needed for developing enough confidence is another matter. Or children might be inclined to fall back more quickly and easily out of habit, or convention or under social pressure, and say they are hungry and thirsty. That would be quite understandable. But basically one can't say that it's no good for children, or diabetics, or convalescents or anyone else. However, as regards global starvation, I don't believe that nourishment through light can be a method of solving this problem for the world.

Question: We have our stomach, our digestive system, our teeth and so on as a gift from God, but you are disregarding this in some way. As someone living in a land of plenty you choose to be nourished by light. But it seems to me that people in poor countries would not be able to exercise such a liberty.

These are important concerns that are justified and should be taken very seriously. By not eating I am of course not contributing in every way possible to God's commandment to Adam: 'Rule over the earth.' I have to try and compensate for this in other ways. If living on light were to lead us to despise physical substance, minerals, plants and so on, this would of course be quite wrong and be damaging rather than helpful. I watch and test myself very thoroughly in this matter and am able to say that since I stopped eating I have cultivated and also newly gained a close relationship to these kingdoms of nature. And as to how I treat my body, I can also tell you about another interesting and presumably typical experience. Since I stopped eating I have gained a noticeably more close, harmonious and loving relationship with my body and am also able to deal with it quite differently. However, no doubt there are also other ways of achieving this.

Regarding the other part of your question: Thousands of

people, mostly children, starve to death every day. But to say: 'There's no need for them to eat, they can live on light', is cynical and smacks of contempt. You can only stop eating when you have had sufficient food to satisfy your hunger. If anything can be done, there may be one possibility, and that would be for people who have enough food to stop eating while ensuring that those who have too little are given some. For me this is thinkable and would be a good and satisfactory way, but I suppose it will remain in the realm of theory.

Question: Do others have a metabolic system that works in the same way, or is this different in every case?
If you are alive your metabolism functions as it must. There's no other possibility. Life is not possible without metabolism. The human body is in a permanent slowly flowing equilibrium or rather non-equilibrium. There must always be some metabolism, if only as a result of breathing. Metabolism can never be brought to a stop for any length of time. There must always be a flowing equilibrium. So one has to assume that there is always more or less the same kind of metabolism, whether a person eats normally or is nourished by light. Logically, however, one must assume that the metabolism we need to live is not necessarily bound up with taking in physical food.

Question: Would you be interested in bringing this subject to public attention on a larger scale through the media?
So long as the media were interested in the subject itself rather than in me as a person I would find this acceptable. If this were the case I would be prepared to collaborate, since I very much hope that the subject of 'living on light' will be given more thought, and that more research will be done and written about it.

Question: Why did you take up 'living on light'? What did you find most fascinating about it?

I suppose it was a good mixture of curiosity, personal circum-stances — since I was rather unwell at the time and hoped it would help me — and a fundamental interest in the esoteric coupled with a sincere wish for self-improvement.

Question: You converted to 'living on light' about four years ago. What are the main changes you have noticed since then?

I have much better health and vitality than before, and I have a more intimate relationship with my body; I appreciate and love it more than I could before. In an agreeable, healthy and natural way I feel more directly and intimately connected with my body. My immune reactions and regenerative forces are noticeably stronger than before. I almost never get ill, and any minor injuries such as are unavoidable in everyday life heal much better and more quickly.

I feel markedly stable emotionally, and mentally enriched since I can concentrate better and my memory is much better than it used to be. On the other hand after converting to 'living on light' I soon noticed that this way of life doesn't work miracles. I am relieved about this because of course I want to remain in charge of my own development and shape it or at least share in shaping it myself.

Question: You said that an essential condition for carrying through the 21-day process was reliance on the thought that you would be nourished by the forces of light whatever happened. Does this mean that you have to be permanently very focused on it?

Not at all. What you have to do is put your trust in that sphere even when there are a thousand logical reasons which speak against this way of receiving nourishment. Nothing much else is necessary. I am convinced that the process of being nourished by light is a gift from the spiritual world which is all around and within us, an endeavour to break through the materialism that is having such a devastating effect just now.

Logical and critical thought should always be present, of course, but these quickly come up against a boundary. Even if you just eat a cheese sandwich and try to understand the resulting digestive processes you soon come to a full stop. Yet they function anyway, you eat and are nourished without entirely understanding how your digestion works. All you need is trust in what is good and helpful.

Question: Do you really believe that light feeds you? What do you think actually nourishes you?
This is a very difficult question to answer. It's very difficult to put it into words. But the term 'living on light' does seem to be the expression that is closest to the truth. Worldwide the word 'light' has positive connotations, for light stands for warmth, strength, illumination and positive evolution. Light is at home at the boundary between the physical and the metaphysical. Many people use other terms to describe the source of the light which gives nourishment, for example cosmic energy, *prana, chi,* the power of Christ, and many others. Really this is just a question of usage or cultural background; it isn't important for the phenomenon as such nor for the actual truth on which it is based.

The process is very intimate and subtle; I experience it as being very positive, very loving, and it inspires confidence.

Question: Would you say something about the difference between fasting and being nourished by light?
When you fast you deprive your body of food and thus of a certain amount of nourishment. The body is then forced to

switch over to using up reserves which it drains, then it begins to deteriorate, and finally you can't go on much longer without something to drink. Normally you fast in order to cleanse the body by shedding what is superfluous, ballast that has accumulated together with toxic substances, thus giving it a good rinse through. But no doubt there are other reasons as well.

The situation is quite different when you have been through the 21-day process and are being nourished by the forces of light. At first it is like fasting, but after three or four days you notice quite clearly that this is no longer fasting. You get a clear impression of once again receiving nourishment.

Question: Personally I find eating and drinking a pleasure. Do you miss something when you abstain? What other pleasures do you go for instead?

I always used to enjoy my food very much, and there are not many sins connected with eating and drinking that I have not committed. Before I started on the 21-day process I weighed 96 kilos [approx. 15 stone] at my heaviest. I had no idea in advance how I would feel without food or whether I would miss anything. But there was virtually no problem. Once in a while I do eat a piece of chocolate or a bit of cheese, or I take a bite out of my children's pizza to tease them, or something like that. But the pleasure of eating anyway ends in one's throat. As soon as you've swallowed the food all that remains is the nuisance factor.

But seriously, I do enormously enjoy being present when people eat, and seeing and smelling the food – like those plates of roasted tomatoes just now in the cafeteria: delicious! And I really do enjoy that. Sometimes I do fancy something, and then I eat a few grapes or nuts, or something else. But I have no trouble doing without food.

Question: I have heard of people embarking on this method and then dying.

Yes, I've read about that too. I know of three cases that have been reported on the internet. Perhaps there have been others. I don't know enough about these to say anything reliable. The small amount of information given made me assume that the starting situation of those people had been problematical and had involved drug abuse in the past, or extreme lifestyles and attitudes. In such situations I would probably have advised waiting for a while. Some measure of stability and self-responsibility should certainly be a precondition.

But on the other hand we need to look at these things in perspective. For example if people are told that a certain diet, or standing on your head for ten minutes every morning, is good for your health, and if perhaps thousands of people do this regularly, then it is likely that on occasion someone might die doing it. Or looked at the other way round: If, which is presumed to be the case, thousands of people have undergone the process of not drinking for seven days and not eating for three weeks, then if three of them have died, this doesn't have all that much to say about the method as such. I'm trying to put the whole thing in proportion and don't mean to talk down the danger. Each one of these cases will have been tragic and dreadful for all those involved. But for the purposes of a risk analysis it is up to every individual to make his or her own judgement.

On the 21-day process

Question: In the book Living on Light *it says that the first few days of the 21-day process are the most difficult, for example that you sweat all the time and feel so overheated that you are virtually forced to do something to cool down. What was your experience?*

As I said just now, you eat and drink nothing during the first few days. Many things can happen as a result, and every case is completely personal and individual. In Jasmuheen's book it says that the first days are very strenuous and that certain symptoms such as sweating and the like can occur. I myself experienced this as a process of cleansing, and I can corroborate most of what she says, including some bouts of feeling weak. These things appear to be necessary, and the early days are the most difficult physiologically. The second week is perhaps psychologically more difficult; the first week is much too strenuous and also too exciting to allow for much in the way of emotional problems. But for me and also some others whom I know personally, the whole of the 21-day process was perfectly manageable.

Question: Is it so that you have to eat ice-cream to cool down, or keep on having to bathe?

One can't generalize about this or exclude other things. Hot flushes are often mentioned, but I didn't experience these. Whatever happens, you have to do whatever is necessary to help yourself in a natural way. I felt cold for a lot of the time and therefore took hot baths. I'm sure common sense will always find a way. I never felt the need to consult a doctor or call for help. And I've never come across this with people I have accompanied through the process either. You mentioned eating ice-cream which of course isn't allowed. But you can chew ice-cubes so long as you don't swallow any of the resulting water.

Question: According to Jasmuheen, a 'heavenly brotherhood' will begin to work in you at the beginning of the fourth day in order to prevent the death processes which would normally commence. Did you experience this consciously and could you describe it?

No, I had no supersensible perceptions of such a process, nor did I directly perceive any higher spiritual being. But during that period I did experience a strong flow of forces from the realm which I, personally, see as being linked to the forces of Christ, and this filled me with joy. I wanted to perceive it more strongly and directly, but instead I slept soundly during the night and only realized in the morning that a definite change had come about. I felt clearly that I was being nourished, and this persists to the present day.

Question: Did you have any clairvoyant or other so-called supersensible experiences during the 21-day process?

I have not become clairvoyant, nor did I have any conscious communication with an angel or anything like that. But I have become noticeably more sensitive. I have a clearly positive basic feeling which was not just an initial burst of euphoria, since it persists to this day. It is a feeling of being on a good path, but I didn't encounter any miracles.

Question: To come back to the question of taking liquids, you mentioned that your body shrivelled rather while you were not drinking anything at all. Could you describe this in more detail?

The fact is that when you are being nourished by light you don't need to drink anything at all. During the conversion phase you are of course very much deprived of liquids, and you begin to dehydrate. Naturally this is also obvious externally at first, and it takes time for your appearance to normalize and for you to become adjusted to the new physical conditions. In the end we are talking about both eating *and* drinking. The aim is to receive *all nourishment* from another source and that means, as I would like to emphasize yet again,

drinking as well as eating. Anything else would be meaningless and to expect it would be illogical.

*Question: Regarding beginning to take liquids after the first
seven days: In the book* Living on Light *it says that one
should not decide oneself when to begin drinking again.
Did you have an inner feeling that told you: 'Now you may
start drinking again'?*

What it says in the book is: Don't drink for 7 days. And 7 days
are 7 times 24 hours. So this is what I did. When undergoing a
conversion process like this I'm sure it's important to avoid
making any arbitrary decisions or those that are based on mood
since this could cause all kinds of completely uncontrollable
things to happen. The book does contain one instruction
regarding the process which is rather unclear, or actually almost
fatal, namely that one can begin to drink again before the 7 days
are up. But it says that one should not decide about this oneself.
Rather, one should only do so if one has an 'impulse' about it
which makes one feel entirely certain. A statement like this can
be rather problematical. I think it's better to play safe and stick
stubbornly, or should I say correctly, to 7 days being 7 times 24
hours. Then if you give the spiritual world the latitude of a few
extra hours you can be sure that everything will be fine.

*Question: Did you go through the process alone or did you
have a mentor?*

Jasmuheen states quite emphatically and clearly that it is not
only advisable but also absolutely necessary to have a personal
mentor during the process, someone you know well, whom you
trust, who knows what you are up to and is willing to keep an
eye on you; if possible a person who has already gone through
the process him or herself. For me the person was a good friend

of my wife on whom I could rely entirely. But apart from this I did the whole thing alone. It wasn't a problem. Nevertheless, I wouldn't advise anyone to have themselves dropped by parachute on to an island in order to have complete peace for the process. And anyway, that isn't necessary.

It's also possible to follow the 21-day process in a group accompanied by someone who has had experience with it. This is on offer every year and is run like a seminar. You have your own room to which you can retire whenever you wish. You can also participate in group conversations and exchange experiences with the others. I'm sure this isn't a bad idea although it wouldn't have suited me personally.

Question: How does your body know that you want to convert to receiving nourishment from light and are not just fasting?
Your body knows because it is wise, in fact much wiser than you are if you allow it to show that it is.

Experiences after the 21-day process

Question: You said earlier that you do quite a lot of sport. How much sport can you do when you're 'living on light'? What about endurance sport?
I'm not what you might call a proper sportsman but I do quite a bit of leisure sport. I play tennis regularly and have discovered that I now play better than before simply because I'm more supple and fitter, and I suppose I react more quickly. Of course a contributory factor is that I've lost quite a bit of weight. But what I find important in this respect is that having converted to a new way of receiving nourishment I have quite a new relationship with my body. I now really enjoy exercise such as walking,

cycling or just running up the stairs. I used to be rather an easy-going type of person, somewhat sluggish, or let's say phlegmatic. However, I don't know what 'living on light' might do for a competitive sportsman. Someone would need to try it out. But I can't imagine it being a real problem.

Question: How much do you sleep compared with before?
I used to sleep a great deal; I loved sleeping good and long. And I always slept very well without having nightmares and suchlike. I would sleep for eight or nine hours and still need my alarm clock to wake up. Now I sleep for five or six hours, wake up without the alarm and immediately feel wide awake, fresh and well rested. And normally this lasts all day. As before, I can rarely remember any dreams.

Question: You said you drink regularly at mealtimes. Do you know of people who don't drink at all?
Yes, there are such people. I try it out from time to time as well, simply because it interests me. I've gone ten days without drinking and felt very well on it. You get a few symptoms to start with, but they're not bad. You also lose a bit of weight and at first your mouth gets dry. That is easily dealt with by cleaning one's teeth or rinsing the mouth. I find that works perfectly well.

Question: How do teeth react when they are no longer used for biting and chewing?
Indeed, one's teeth no longer have much to do. I've been to the dentist several times, and once I also had trouble with a filling. I haven't told my dentist anything, and he hasn't noticed — or anyway he hasn't made any remarks. In other words, there's nothing unusual. Naturally I had been rather worried about my teeth. People say that it isn't good for the teeth when they have

nothing to bite, or for example when you choose a diet that requires very little chewing, because chewing is like a massage for the gums. It is said that teeth start to wobble and threaten to fall out. But I can't corroborate this. My teeth have so far behaved perfectly normally – even though I don't chew on a bone as a substitute...

Question: Do your teeth in fact improve as a result of living on light?
That I can't say yet. But in the daytime one's mouth and jaws still get a certain amount of exercise simply through speaking. The body is wise enough not to let things go rusty so long as one doesn't prevent it. And surely this also applies to the teeth. It seems that these things are self-regulating in a natural way. I'm not aware of any problem. I clean my teeth regularly and frequently. I do it thoroughly and enjoy doing so because it feels good. Perhaps that is all that's needed.

Question: If a pregnant woman lives on light and then her child is born, is her breast-milk superfluous?
Mother's milk surely has many important functions. There's the warmth, the bodily contact, love; it isn't purely physical food. I don't know whether you can say it's all superfluous. If you can compensate for all the other things, then perhaps mother's milk is superfluous for building up the child's physical body. Perhaps it's theoretically possible, but I don't know. If you think logically it might be the case, but for now this is total supposition.

Question: You said you sometimes eat a few grapes or nuts or something like that. Is this good or bad?
And: You have a family. How do they react? Have they accepted your conversion?

Interestingly enough, my 'little lapses' now no longer present any problems. But formerly I also never had any problems with my digestion. Of course it all depends on the amount, what it is you eat, and the circumstances. So long as you are more or less sensible there's no need to worry. Of course if you were in my situation I wouldn't recommend sauerkraut with pigs' trotters. That would certainly be too much. There is, after all, finally a limit to how much flexibility can be coped with. But a little bit of something is evidently not a problem.

As to your second question: My family have grown accustomed to my behaviour, but it certainly did take some getting used to. I have done my best already to emphasize this very important aspect of the social awkwardness that arises in connection with 'living on light'. Really this cannot be stressed too often. If there is any problem at all in connection with 'living on light', then it's the matter of how to deal with one's social environment. This is the biggest problem and one that has to be handled sensitively, with care and as much awareness as possible. Anyone intending to undertake the conversion must be fully clear about this. It is often underestimated, but as I have shown, it can be coped with quite well.

Question: If you perspire heavily, in the summer or from exertion, do you feel thirsty, or has this also diminished with time?

In winter I go to the sauna at regular intervals where I certainly perspire a lot, which I find very agreeable. After that my mouth is dry and I have a drink of something. However, if you didn't want to drink I think you could probably get away with rinsing your mouth and cleaning your teeth.

Question: I have read that you work in a company with other colleagues. Is there a problem of not being taken seriously or causing amusement?

As I have stressed many times before: if there is a problem, then it is a social one. Many people do find it difficult to deal with the fact that someone, perhaps whom they know well and esteem, suddenly no longer eats food. I always held back, and normally still do, with regard to telling people about how I receive nourishment, especially when I'm not directly asked. This has been a good policy and one I can recommend wholeheartedly. At my workplace the time did arrive when I had to 'come out of the closet' and tell my colleagues about my new way of life, which I then did openly and honestly and with modesty. Since then all my colleagues have got used to the idea, so that there is no longer a problem and the subject never gets mentioned – seeing as I don't work as a chef, or a food taster...

Question: So you have no medical problems and even claim that you feel better than before? Is there no kind of disadvantage for the physical body?

Of course I can only speak for myself, and I don't think it would be a good idea to generalize. 'Living on light' is not a panacea that can solve all physical problems. This would be an entirely false conclusion and one that could lead to much disappointment and frustration. However, the fact is that in my case I have not noticed any disadvantages with this way of life but rather only the advantages already mentioned. I feel much more healthy and energetic physically, more stable emotionally, and mentally more sure of myself, more alert and fit.

Question: We also take in nourishment through our senses. Have you noticed whether your sense organs are more awake, whether you feel you can take in and experience things through your senses more intensely than before?

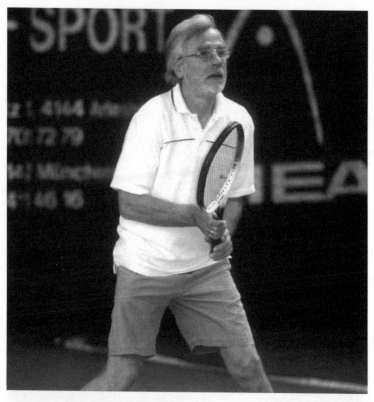

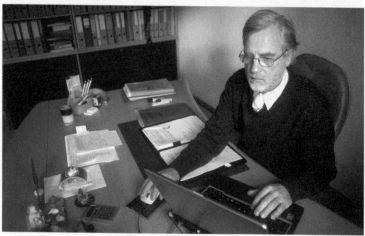

Michael Werner: Regular exercise for fun; everyday work at the office.

That is definitely the case. It even happens with ordinary fasting. You become more sensitive, indeed often oversensitive and nervy. This is a very important point that should be mentioned. There are many methods that can be used to increase one's sensitivity. There's nothing wrong with this in principle, but it can be somewhat ticklish. Refinement of one's sensitivity should always go hand in hand with a corresponding degree of increased inner stability. Sensitivity is only good if a person is also inwardly stable. Those who are too sensitive but insufficiently stable are likely to end up in a mental hospital. Psychiatric clinics are full of such people, and this is a great tragedy. Personally I can say that I haven't found being nourished by light a danger in this respect, not even during the 21-day process. I feel markedly stable, and for me this has always been an important yardstick to apply in deciding whether I am ready to proceed with something. If this had not been the case I would have abandoned the 'experiment' long ago, since the price would have been far too high and the matter too dangerous.

Question: I was surprised to hear you say that you have become more closely connected with your body since you gave up eating. Normally if you reduce the amount you eat or when you begin an ordinary fast there's more of a danger of becoming less firmly connected with your body. You cause the ties between body, sense-perceptions, emotions and the mental sphere to loosen.

It is definitely surprising and unexpected that there is such good bodily stability when one is being nourished by light despite the fact that with ordinary fasting one's stability tends to decrease. However, we should be aware of a misunderstanding which we must be very clear about. We need to draw a distinction between food and receiving nourishment. It is one thing to stop eating solid food. And if in consequence one is not being nourished, then one loses one's stability, and this can quickly become a problem. But if one has converted to being nourished by light and has opened oneself to the forces of light, then one can be adequately nourished without eating physical food in the usual way, and in that case there is not necessarily any loss of stability.

Question: What about bad breath after the 21-day process?
Of course the problem is familiar to me. It happens frequently with any change of diet – almost always when cleansing processes are taking place within the body – even without the 21-day process. When it arises you have to find your own individual solution. Perhaps you need to clean your teeth more often or suck a peppermint from time to time. Of course the latter mustn't be done during the 21-day process which requires strictly no eating and no drinking – since a peppermint remains a peppermint. But afterwards it's perfectly alright to suck a sweet. It's up to the individual.

Question: You said you drink regularly. How do you relate to coffee, water, juice, wine and suchlike? And how was it at first and how is it now?
As I said, I drink something when I'm with people who are having a meal, and what I drink depends on the occasion. Among other things coffee – which is available almost anywhere – fruit juice, water, sometimes a glass of wine. I don't drink for any particular reason or with some purpose in mind, and also not because I'm thirsty. I drink to be sociable, but I could also simply not drink anything at all.

As a general rule I get up in the morning and have a cup of coffee or two at breakfast with my family. At work I have an espresso for elevenses with my colleagues. At lunchtime I might have a glass of water or juice, or something else. And in the afternoon, perhaps when I'm at a meeting, I may have another coffee. This varies quite a bit, but the amount I drink in a day is somewhere between a litre and a litre and a half. At weekends, perhaps if I go sailing, I might drink very little or even nothing. It depends what comes up, really.

Metabolism and food

Question: I should like to know more about cell metabolism which involves the elimination of used substances to enable new cells to be formed so that over time a complete renewal takes place. Are new cells formed as the result of 'living on light'?

Cell metabolism definitely takes place. I have had readings of my cell metabolism taken several times, and they are more or less normal. My breathing has also been tested, and my respiratory ratio, i.e. the ratio of oxygen to carbon dioxide in the inhaled and exhaled air, is also perfectly normal. This shows that I have a normal cell metabolism which arises at the end of the food chain and is therefore measurable. The question is, though, where does it begin? Where do the 'raw materials' come from? There must be a condensation leading to the initial substances or raw materials. Whether this is really the case and what the physiological details of the process are, I don't know, and I presume no one does.

Question: What is the situation with vitamins, minerals, and trace elements, some of which are seen as being essential for life?

In the eyes of modern physiology no nutritional requirement is either more or less necessary for life than any other. In the final analysis everything belongs together, so that if something is missing which is normally present in abundance, deficiencies will arise and things will soon start to go wrong.

However, in relation to receiving nourishment from light this is the wrong question to ask. Either you can 'live on light' or you cannot. It's illogical to say that 'living on light' is possible if you then also say that as there won't be any selenium or vitamin B_{12} intake these will have to be given separately.

Question: What happens to the digestive tract as a whole when no food is ingested, and how does excretion take place?

Some excretion takes place, for example in urine, sweat and exhaled air. I kept a detailed account of my urine for quite a long time. The amount of urine excreted is 80 to 90 per cent of the daily amount I drink. There is very little excretion of solids: once a week about the amount produced by a rabbit. This presumably arises because cells are shed by the intestinal surface, and perhaps the body accumulates the small amount of fibre in fruit juices. During the 10 days of the scientific study,* when I drank diluted tea at first and then only mineral water, I had no solid motions. My intestines were X-rayed repeatedly and found to be completely void.

As to the digestive organs that have become redundant, such as the stomach, intestines, liver, gall bladder and so on: I find this is not a problem and there is no sign of regression. The readings taken also show there has been no degeneration. When people fast, on the other hand, it is known that the digestive organs regress as time goes on, presumably not from lack of activity but from a lack of nourishment which leads to a kind of 'self-digestion', 'auto-cannibalism' that ultimately ends in death.

---

* See pages 132–154.

When the nourishment comes from light this is fundamentally different. I experience my everyday condition as being in a kind of 'stand-by' mode. Although not functioning, the whole system is intact. The only explanation must be that as before the organs are receiving normal and sufficient sustenance, only in a different way. This is what all the laboratory tests done to date have shown in the main. There is no deprivation, no deficiency. I sense and experience this condition as I otherwise did between meals or after digestion had taken place, and this is presumably what it is.

Question: Would you be able to eat a helping of spaghetti today if you felt like it?
I am sure that I can begin eating again whenever I want. As I just said, my body and especially my digestive organs feel like they used to feel between meals. By this I mean that the digestive organs are in a kind of resting mode in which they are ready to begin reacting and working as before.

Question: You said that you began the conversion process when you were rather overweight and that your weight is now stable. Do all people who try the process lose weight as a matter of course?
It seems that people virtually always lose weight during the first week of the 21-day process. The amount varies and presumably depends on how overweight or underweight they are in the first place. I have met individuals who were obviously underweight, but they still lost 4 or 5 kilos during the first week. Later on this evens out.

Question: Are you consciously aware that you are being nourished and supported by light energy?
When I take my general sense of wellbeing together with the fact that I am receiving energy and nourishment from light in the

way described, then I can say that I am certainly aware of this, but not in the sense that I suddenly get the feeling: I need some light now, or some food from light. The process of energy supply and the conversion of matter seems to carry on evenly or, if it really kicks in when there is an actual need, then so gently that I personally am not aware of it.

Question: In order to determine the basal conversion, you measure the amount of oxygen taken in and of carbon dioxide given out and make a calculation which shows that the body is functioning normally in a way that can be checked. I simply can't explain this in your case. Surely you are constantly losing water; that is unavoidable. The calculation could perhaps work out at an air humidity of 100 per cent, when as much water would be going in as coming out.

Such questions remain open at present although many of them could be explained or at least tackled meaningfully by the methods now available to medical research. The scientific pre-conditions are certainly already given. My basal energy conversion has already been measured, by the way, and was found to be completely normal. But scientists have only just begun researching and perhaps even explaining the phenomena and the paradoxes that prevail in this connection.

Question: When a person hasn't eaten for a while they usually feel hungry. Don't you have any sense of being satisfied or hungry?

Actually I feel neither the one nor the other. I'm not satisfied in the sense of feeling replete and wanting to rest a bit while I digest. But neither does my tummy rumble hungrily while I wonder when the next meal will be ready. But I remember both these sensations very well, and sometimes they reappear quite naturally in my emotions. It's not that I don't care about food; indeed I enjoy very much being in the company of people who are eating. Feeling what it's like to eat is very agreeable and gives me much pleasure.

Question: In Rudolf Steiner's lectures on agriculture* there is one in which he described an interplay between cosmic and physical food and nourishment and pointed out that bodily substance is built up via respiration and light and can enter into the tissues at whatever point it is needed.
Steiner gave a good many interesting and helpful hints which I shall not repeat just now (see p. 165). For example he spoke in some detail about what he called a subtle silica process which takes place via the sense organs and brings substance into the body. This also happens via respiration and the skin.

Question: What is the difference between anorexia and your way of receiving nourishment?
A typical anorexic has a negative relationship with the body and with food as such. On the other hand I am very comfortable in my body and feel even closer to it than I did before. And I also still have a very positive attitude towards food and eating. It is a pleasure for me to be present at mealtimes and I often think that I now enjoy meals even more than I would if I had to eat them!

Questions of science

Question: I was astonished to hear that it was necessary for a foundation to promise funding before a scientific investigation of your case could be undertaken [see p. 133].

---

* R. Steiner, 1993.

I would have expected there to be quite a scramble to get hold of you once you knocked at the door of a university hospital. You would expect the portals of science to be thrown wide open to someone who says he has not eaten anything for years, wouldn't you?

All I can say is that this definitely doesn't happen. In fact most medics and physiologists have absolutely no interest in investigating the phenomenon. Having gained quite a bit of experience in this field I could tell you a good many horror stories about it. I have no idea what exactly goes on in the minds of experts. I used to think as you do, but I was wrong. It simply isn't the case.

Question: Where or how do you believe that light energy is transformed into matter or cells in your body?

I can't say, since I have no direct experience of it. I just don't know. It seems possible that it goes on all over the body all the time. Perhaps in the walls of the intestines, or in the lymph flowing towards the liver, or in the liver itself. Perhaps also in the blood. I really don't know. Perhaps the way you have put the question is wrong in the sense that maybe the very nature of the process makes it impossible to fix in space and time. I find these questions extremely exciting. They are not only interesting but also very important for the future. That's why I am quite annoyed at the lack of interest in scientific quarters.

Question: You say you are going to submit to an experiment in which you are under permanent observation. How is the research question framed? What would be the best result? How will the world react to it?

Neither my own questions nor those of the study director, a good friend of mine, a medical doctor, could be so directly included in the design of the study. It had to be formulated in a way that would be acceptable both to the university hospital and the ethics commission. Both these bodies are basically convinced that this whole thing doesn't tie up, since something can't be possible if it isn't allowed! For someone to turn up and say that he remains perfectly healthy even though he no longer eats is an impossibility. We all know from much research that when a person stops eating a great many changes immediately take place in the blood, for example the triglycerides (keto bodies), blood sugar, cholesterol, certain minerals and so on. And the same goes for the urine. Most of these changes are predictable, as we know from many studies, for example in cases of fasting. So these parameters first have to be investigated in this experiment. In other words the study is not in the first instance interested in proving that being nourished by light works. And anyway this cannot be expected of a study lasting only ten days. So it will be a matter of showing that something is going on here which shouldn't actually be happening and can't be expected to happen. Our hope is that this study will open a door so that perhaps in a second step, within the framework of another study, experiments will be undertaken which go into the matter more deeply. This would be an initial step towards acceptance of the phenomenon as such, a phenomenon that is worth researching.

Meditation and other exercises as preparation

Question: You have described in a very relaxed manner how you converted to a new way of receiving nourishment and what happened when you did it. Did you just begin to do it one day, or did you work at it in advance from the other angle as well, from the spiritual aspect? I find it quite difficult to accept your relaxed attitude.

It will be difficult to answer your question because all these things are relative. I can only describe my own experience, and I try to do this as honestly and comprehensibly as possible. Of course every picture has its limitations because it is subjective. So it isn't much help to say that analytical psychology was involved, or teachings on reincarnation or whatever else. We always have a limited pattern of ourselves as well as of others. For example I was very surprised to hear about the possibility of living entirely on light. I wasn't on the lookout for such an idea and didn't say: At last I've found it! It simply came to me as information. But then I decided quite quickly to do it or at least to find out about it. But in my experience you can't generalize about these things. Perhaps it was my destiny, for whatever reason. But it was definitely not the case that I had to make conscious efforts to understand it in order to ensure that the thing would work well, or would even work at all. I simply said to myself one day: This business of 'living on light' – I'm going to do it. To be honest, I do sometimes tend to be somewhat rash or hasty in the way I deal with seeming problems. Anyway, this is how I did it, and I have so far not regretted my decision for a moment.

Question: I believe everything you have told us, and you have succeeded in describing it all clearly and comprehensibly. But I have to say that I do find it difficult when I hear that it is only a question of belief and trust. When you think of so many children and babies starving to death every day, surely one should try and find a collective way of thinking that could bring help to them.

I do understand very well what you are saying. And it goes not only for the countless children in Africa or Asia but also for many people here in our own country. If they stop eating, or don't get anything to eat, or don't want to eat, they too will starve. This is a dogma that has been drummed into us by education, by our culture and by our religion. Normally and quite naturally we are convinced that if we don't eat anything we will unavoidably die. This generates an environment of causes and effects that leads to our starvation. There must be a breakthrough in this, and there can be a breakthrough.

Question: At this point I now have another question on the matter of belief. You mentioned that one must be open, must open oneself. When I think about what you mean I try to open myself through meditation and in other ways. But I don't know whether I am reaching that inmost complex, my own supersensible organism so that I can truly open myself to the forces of light. I do think that I believe, which as you said is the most important precondition for the process if it is to function. But if I were to do it without believing, then it wouldn't work; I can well imagine this and feel that it's right. Yet if I think that I believe, but if there is a doubter hidden deep inside me who is convinced that I need physical food in order to live, then I can also well imagine that it won't work. This is what seems to me to be the ability and also the actual difficulty.

In this connection I would like to add another component to the idea of believing, and that is trust. What you seem to mean is that to believe something also means not to know it.

Believing is an important precondition for making the 21-day process and the nourishment by light that follows it work, so that one doesn't after all die of hunger or thirst. But as I have just said, trust also plays a very important part in this. We trust that this form of receiving nourishment conforms with our wishes, and thereupon it does indeed conform with them of its own accord. That is why the possible doubts that still lurk somewhere in us are not such a problem. In fact they are rather normal. Doubt and trust do not cancel one another out, but they can alternate. I am saying this because I remember it all only too well. I went through the process and kept saying to myself: 'It is going to work. Ingrid did it and it worked, so I can try it too, and it'll work. But anyway, if it doesn't work then I'll simply stop and begin eating again. At least I'll then know that it doesn't work.' I certainly had some reservations and was ready to stop if something didn't seem quite right during the process. Nevertheless, you do have to have that fundamental openness as well so as not to be closed up. If you had the attitude that expected it not to work, then that would definitely be a problem.

Question: Is there a way of practising the kind of trust you mention? Or is it a question of courage? Is it only something for the chosen few, or even a gift for them only?
I have nothing specific to say about that. You must have trust, or you must develop it. You also need to have trust in yourself. And if you lack courage you have to take it from somewhere.

Question: I believe it's something you feel in yourself. You feel it and then you want to do it. Just as you knew directly that you wanted to go through the conversion process.
Yes, that is a good and important point. I think you sense it and then you know exactly that you want to do it or that you should do it or are permitted to do it. This is something important: I think that those who follow the process sense that it is for them. Jasmuheen put it very beautifully in her book: 'When your heart begins to sing, then you go through this process.' That's a right and beautiful way of putting it.

Question: Do you ask to be fed by the light?
Yes, I ask for it, and again and again I feel very grateful for it.

Question: You mentioned that you had had health problems before deciding to convert to living on light. Do you think that there are some illnesses with health risks of a kind that would make it unwise to embark on such a conversion?
I don't have anything concrete to say with regard to the risks. I don't know if they are relevant. But I'm sure that a diabetic, or someone with kidney problems, would take this into account by being especially careful and circumspect when approaching the conversion.

Question: How do you tune in to the power of the light? Are there any special meditations for this?
For many years I have been cultivating a very personal and intensive meditative life which I have always felt to be enriching and a help even in everyday life. Since I had already had the practice of setting aside certain intervals during the day for meditation which enriched my life and influenced it in positive ways, I don't know how things would have gone without such meditation. But I have a feeling that if you open yourself trustingly to the process of receiving nourishment from light everything will run of its own accord.

Question: What spiritual development have you undertaken, and how have you changed in other ways since your conversion to 'living on light'?
I listen to a lot of music. I specially like Mozart and Beethoven for instance. I read many books and do quite a few other things for which I had no time before. I am not clairvoyant, but I sense that

I am following a good path. Psychologically I feel more stable and sensitive than before and altogether richer. I find I am much more able to have good thoughts and feelings than previously, and I look to the future with much optimism and confidence.

3
On the 21-day process
by Thomas Stöckli based on Charmaine Harley

We have already referred several times to the process which was first described in the book *Living on Light* by Jasmuheen and thereafter became known around the world as the 21-day process. Although one is inclined to regard the book itself with a critical eye on account of its being a somewhat 'esoteric miscellany', Michael Werner has always stressed that the description of the 21-day process itself is basically very helpful and indeed essential for anyone wanting to convert to living on light. But one must realize that as an 'instruction manual' the book itself should be treated with some caution since the risks and dangers inherent in the conversion process are only mentioned explicitly by Jasmuheen in her follow-up volume.

Let us, however, not throw the baby out with the bath-water. There are individuals everywhere who, in remaining true to themselves, follow their own path in their search for the truth, so it is just as inappropriate to condemn out of hand every New Age exponent as it is to become a naive camp-follower. As mentioned earlier, Michael Werner has never met Jasmuheen but he regards her as a pioneer working to open up new spiritual horizons, even though he by no means agrees with all she has to say.

The following brief summary and overview of the 21-day process is included here because of its central importance in working towards receiving nourishment from light. It must not be taken as a complete set of instructions and is not intended as a substitute for the full description contained in Jasmuheen's book. So anyone seriously seeking further information and guidance should definitely consult the original book.

The origin of the 21-day process

The 21-day process explains how to convert from an ordinary diet to living on light. It first appeared in Australia in the late autumn of 1992, mediated by a medium via the method of channelling, which means that it is a direct communication and information coming from a spiritual sphere. It is assumed that the process was first practised by some individuals and then passed on telepathically to others. Jasmuheen was not one of the first to practise it, but having come across the information early in 1993 she has since then been spreading the word energetically. She is supported in this by her own experience and ability as a medium using channelling.

Her book *Living on Light* was published in 1996 and it generated a wave of interest all around the world. It was translated into German in 1997 and then brought out again in English in 1998 as *Living on Light, The Source of Nourishment for the New Millennium*. The description of the 21-day process takes up about 45 of the book's 200 pages. The most important information, however, is not formulated and written by Jasmuheen but by Charmaine Harley who followed the conversion process in June 1994 and subsequently compiled her recommendations and suggestions. These were initially distributed in Australia in pamphlet form. We regard them as the standard instruction for following the path to becoming nourished by light.

One must always emphasize, however, that these are only guidelines. We expressly recommend that individuals should apply their own faculties of discrimination and listen to their own inner guide. The descriptions and statements do not explain everything, and are indeed not intended to be exhaustive.

Charmaine Harley's suggestions and recommendations for the 21-day process are presented in two parts, dealing first with basic information on how to prepare and then describing the process as such in detail. We present our compilation of the most important statements in the following.

Preparing for the process

An essential tool to help decide on and prepare for the process is provided in a 15-point self-screening questionnaire. One should be able honestly to say Yes to all the questions. They are intended to help a person decide whether this moment is right and meaningful as the starting point for the process. One should know from within oneself whether one will be capable of carrying it through, and the process should be regarded as a 'sacred initiation'. It is important to be willing to accept and follow a few rules regarding eating and drinking for the whole three week period.

Having decided to enter into the process, the next thing to be done is to set out an exact schedule with the intention of adhering to it. It is also important to organize one's personal and social circumstances in a way that will leave one free and relaxed during the process. The small details of everyday life and routine responsibilities should be taken care of in advance or organized to impinge as little as possible during the 21 days.

If possible one should find a care-giver who has already undergone the process and who is willing to be available during it. As far as is possible, everything should be discussed and clarified with this person in advance of beginning the process. It is advisable to prepare the body and indeed also oneself to enable the transition to be as easy as may be and a source of joy.

In practical terms this means: In the run-up to beginning, stop eating meat if possible, and perhaps change over to raw food entirely, and in the last few days perhaps have only soup and other liquids. At least in the final three days alcohol should be avoided, and this as well as drugs and tobacco are of course quite unsuitable for the duration of the three weeks.

'Be prepared for a period of solitude. It is a sacred and precious time and it would be unfortunate if you were prevented by difficult outer circumstances from enjoying and appreciating the process.'

Throughout the process the essential element is not a matter of whether one eats or does not eat but of knowing that higher levels of energy can be tapped in such a way that one no longer needs any physical food.

Going through the process

It is emphatically recommended to include two helpers. First a care-giver is needed who lives nearby and can supply practical assistance — someone who, so to speak, lends physical support. This person bears a heavy responsibility, for the task calls for love, understanding, willingness to be involved, sensitivity, strength and, of course, mutual trust. There should be daily visits from this person to provide physical care and to ensure that the necessary peace and quiet can be maintained, with all unnecessary distractions and stress kept at bay so that one can be relaxed and devoted to oneself and turn one's attention towards the spiritual world. The second person functions as a mentor and should also have undergone the process in order to give support out of personal experience if reassurance and help are required.

One should be ready for three weeks of nothing worldly, no television, no phone, computer, noise, stress, family or social obligations, fixed dates, appointments, obligations (garden, pets etc.), so as to be able to devote oneself as far as possible to the process itself. One should also consider whether it might be better to desist from one's usual physical and mental exercises (e.g. yoga or meditation) for the duration of the conversion process.

It is important that one's surroundings should be as pleasant and stress-free as possible. The requirement is for peace, comfort, warmth, much light and fresh air and easy access to nice walks. Prepare to have good, light reading and beautiful music available as well as fruit juices and water in sufficient quantities.

One strong recommendation is to keep a detailed diary.

As the process continues, various symptoms of bodily and psychological cleansing can occur, such as are known to those who have tried out fasting cures. Among these are headaches, coated tongue, halitosis, nausea, sleeplessness, bad mood, irritability and restlessness. These symptoms of detoxification are usually bearable and on the whole not a cause for concern.

The process

The 21-day process consists of three 7-day phases. It thereby follows age-old sacred and healing rhythms of time. The instructions differ for each of these phases:

The first 7 days

You neither eat nor drink.

This is the period during which the actual conversion takes place when the necessary cleansing process comes about.

It should be a time of rest and quiet when you can be entirely within yourself.

On the second day you may have 'fasting symptoms' such as headache, kidney pains, muscular pains, and coated mucous membranes. You may feel groggy, weak and a bit 'wobbly' on your legs.

You may relieve your thirst only by rinsing your mouth or chewing ice-cubes and then spitting out any liquid.

During the night from the third to the fourth day a decisive change takes place, a transformation which in some instances is clearly experienced but in others passes unnoticed and is only perceived the following morning. The need for the body to transform itself can sometimes lead to a sensation of emptiness, but many people do not experience this directly.

In the days that follow there is still no eating or drinking allowed. Peace and relaxation are needed for the process of reorientation to take place. You might feel groggy or weak, have erratic, hectic thoughts, or lack feeling. Some are nervous and irritable, and you may experience hot flushes. These processes should be followed with trust and gratitude, and without anxiety.

During the late afternoon or evening of the seventh day you may drink a little for the first time. The moment when this takes place should be discussed with your mentor. If you are in doubt or feel inwardly uncertain, wait until the end of the seventh day before you drink.

The second 7 days

Peace, relaxation, healing and cleansing are the main themes during the second week. This should be a wonderful time which you enjoy in peace and quiet even if you feel somewhat weak and fragile.

Still nothing is eaten, but water or orange juice (diluted to 25 per cent concentration), a minimum of one-and-a-half litres per day, is allowed. The fluid serves to cleanse the body and stabilize the changes that have taken place in the first week. You will have a sense of energy flowing into you.

How a person feels during these days varies from individual to individual. You may feel anxious and unwell or even ill, or have an extreme sense of being full of energy.

The third 7 days

Still you may not eat, but you may drink. Fruit juices diluted to 40 per cent concentration are allowed and indeed recommended. You begin to feel stronger and therefore more 'normal'. The good feeling of being on your way to a new life and the sense that you are becoming more stable each day will give you courage and strength.

As a rule the process is complete at the end of the twenty-first day. You are now being nourished and maintained, it is said, by 'prana' or 'light' or energies from the 'etheric' realm of creation.

After completing the 21-day process

You return to everyday life after 21 days having accomplished an unusual journey in which you have changed much. Everything is still in flux and there is much to which you will have to accustom yourself. Some people have an unfamiliar yet pleasant and liberating sense of detachment, and in general there is a definite increase of sensitivity in one's sense perceptions. Healing and stabilizing processes are still in progress, so you are well advised to take good care of yourself in the coming days and weeks. Be considerate to yourself and live cautiously even if the changes are not immediately obvious. If at all possible, prolong the free and quiet time by bringing the 21-day process to an end in a gradual way.

You can now make you own decisions about how you want to live, since there is no longer any physiological need for you to eat and drink. But you are perfectly free to do so if you wish. Any wish to drink or eat solid food that may arise from now on will have an emotional or mental origin. You should treat these wishes gently and give yourself time to decide on definitive and absolute changes on the basis of your personal situation. If you want to continue taking liquids, you are entirely free to decide what, how and how much you want to drink.

As to participating in the usual meals with your family, with friends or your wider social set-up, there are few reasons why you should not do so but many why you should if you so wish. Experience has shown that drinking something while the others eat is a good way of distracting attention from the fact that you are not eating, and it also means that the others at the table will be less embarrassed.

It is important to be aware that the instructions about eating and drinking apply absolutely only to the three weeks of the process. It is up to the person to choose which, if any, of the other suggestions and recommendations he or she wishes to take up. One can and should adapt one's decisions to the personal, individual situation and to one's own needs and aspirations. And in the last resort one should always listen to the inner voice of feelings and conscience.

Personal reports on following the 21-day process

Michael Werner spends a great deal of time corresponding at length on the subject of 'living on light' and has repeatedly also accompanied individuals through the conversion process if he sensed that they were genuinely embarking on it on their own responsibility and had not been influenced by others in reaching their decision to do so.

In the final analysis there are, in fact, relatively few people who feel called upon to undertake this venture. We should here stress once again that certain preconditions must be met in order to avoid unnecessary damage to one's health or other difficulties. Although conversion might appear to be rather a matter of course in the way Michael Werner has described it, nevertheless, depending on the initial situation, it can be risky; damage could arise if this form of receiving nourishment were to be encouraged in an irresponsible manner. It is essential to take the decision to go ahead on one's own responsibility, to make careful preparations and, in most cases, to be accompanied by a person whom one trusts and who has had experience of living on light.

The following reports by people who have gone through the 21-day process have been selected to demonstrate how very different the great variety of personal experiences can be and also to show the kind of problem that can arise both during the process and after its completion.

In addition the reports show that living on light can be considered not only in isolated, exceptional cases but also by perfectly ordinary individuals. The reader will gain an impression of the many and varied ways in which it can be tackled and will also become acquainted with the many further possibilities involved. The fairly random bunch of personal accounts and individual opinions presented here has arisen out of the necessity to select or rather reduce the number of examples that could be cited.

All the reports come from individuals known personally to Michael Werner. Some of them have connections with anthroposophy, which arose naturally from the fact that Michael Werner himself is connected with this way of thinking and because the first detailed report on him was published in the German-language weekly journal of the Anthroposophical Society, *Das Goetheanum*. However, this does not necessarily mean that any cogent connection should be inferred.

Report by Benno Walbeck

I first learned about the 21-day process in the autumn of 2002 from an article in the journal *Das Goetheanum*. I had just turned 39 and was in the twelfth year of working as a teacher. Both my children were living with their mother from whom I was divorced. The separation had been difficult in every respect. I was living alone, had just moved to another town and was trying to find my feet in my new surroundings.

Initially I was surprised that *Das Goetheanum* would publish such an article since it seemed to me that the literature quoted and the process as such could not be compatible with anthroposophy. But the editors evidently felt it would be important for their readers. I myself was immediately attracted to the process described. I did not doubt that one could live on light and straight away I asked myself: Is it really possible for anyone to do this — even me?

I was convinced that I wanted to try it out. But on the other hand something in me also felt repelled. As a young person I had considered taking up farming because working with the land had seemed to me to be one of the great needs of our time. Would such tasks now become redundant? I couldn't imagine that. And if it were to be possible for everyone to live on light, would that call into question the hitherto irrefutable dogma 'three days without water, a few weeks without bread, and you'll be dead', the implication being that people die of thirst or hunger simply because this is what they expect. I would have found such an idea exceedingly unsettling.

Not long after reading the article I met Michael Werner and attended one of his lectures about living on light. So I became more familiar with the subject, though as some questions were cleared up new ones arose. I began to realize that living on light would not solve the problem of feeding the world, since the decision to take it up is entirely a matter for the individual which cannot be decided by others. My own wish to try it out for myself grew as time went on.

About a year after hearing about it I embarked on the 21-day process. Apart from being curious as to whether I would really be capable of living on light, I was also motivated by other considerations such as having more time, more energy and better health, and easing the pressure on my budget.

I encountered many obstacles, often from unexpected quarters. The first difficulty was deciding on a date, since it would be difficult for me to withdraw from my everyday life for three weeks. There was no question of using the summer holidays, but the other periods free of teaching were only two weeks long, and being a teacher meant that I couldn't choose to take time off except during those times. After putting the whole thing off twice

I finally decided to convert during the 16 days of the autumn break while having to accept that the first three days and the final two would impinge on working time. I have always engaged in a good deal of sport, so my physical condition was good. Having talked this timing through with the mentor who was to accompany me through the process, we agreed that it would be possible.

I went through the process at home with a helper living in. My mentor telephoned regularly and also dropped by for chats. I was not too strict with the book's instructions regarding spending most of the time alone. But I kept firmly to the daily regime of alternating periods of rest and activity, and to the instructions about drinking (nothing for the first seven days, and a lot for the following 14). Neither hunger nor thirst bothered me much, but I had difficulties with my dry mouth (which I didn't want to rinse) and with having to spend so much time lying down. Having neither a balcony nor a patch of garden I missed natural surroundings. I got someone to drive me out and accompany me on my daily walks. Towards the end of the first week I felt dizzy and weak when walking. Apart from this I achieved the conversion without any problems worth mentioning. Talks with my mentor were very helpful, since questions arose which were not dealt with in the book.

I was astonished by how relatively well I managed without drinking. My greatest worry had been whether doing what I intended to do would be life-threatening, and I had decided to break off the process if I detected any signs of danger. But I had absolutely no kidney pain, which is supposed to be a sign of lack of fluid intake.

Among the many changes and peculiarities I experienced there were four which stood out most clearly:

— I woke up at around 4 o'clock every morning having had enough sleep, and I continued to have a much reduced need for sleep.

— I was able to concentrate on my work for noticeably longer periods.

— When my helper was cooking for himself he apologized for the smells. I meanwhile inhaled them greedily without having any desire to eat. On the contrary, the thought of tasting food nauseated me.

— Six months previously, I had had to take time off because of serious problems with varicose veins. The veins now disappeared entirely.

When I went back to work people noticed that I had changed. After all, I had lost nearly 10 kilos in weight and my face also looked thinner. My class (ninth year) heard rumours about what I had been up to and expressed a wish to talk to me about it. I arranged a time and they all came except one who was already familiar with the subject. The pupils' main concerns were: Is it really possible to live on light? How do you do it? Why are you doing it? And they reacted in various ways: disbelief (It's impossible); uncertainty (Surely it isn't possible, but why would he lie to us?); acceptance (It's exciting, I think it's great that he's doing it); disapproval (No doubt it's possible, but how can he bring himself to do it?). Some colleagues also made remarks (How can you teach without eating anything?) but they never initiated any conversation.

In the early days the whole thing was something of a sensation at school. Many pupils approached me about it, which was not always agreeable, but there were also humorous episodes. For example a birthday present was to be gift vouchers for sessions at a solarium, or on being invited to a meal I was asked did I prefer to 'eat' 40 or 60 Watts. But I was also closely watched and everything I did was critically assessed. Whatever I did or said raised comments such as: So this is how someone speaks or acts who no longer eats anything. Any reaction of mine that the pupils didn't like was quickly put down to my being in a bad mood again: No wonder, if you never eat! For my part I didn't feel that my moods were any worse than before. No matter what the reason, anything I did was always attributed to not eating, with no account being given to any other possible motivations.

After a while people got used to me and the sensation died down. Although reactions to my conversion had sometimes been hard to bear, my overall feeling was always one of wellbeing. My expectations had been fulfilled and sometimes even exceeded. Initially, for example, I found it quite difficult to handle all the extra time I had, since the complete absence of the need to shop, cook and wash up saves a great deal of time when you live alone. Eating as a social occupation posed more of a problem. Grandma enjoys baking a cake for her grandson, and friends invite you to a meal. Everyone was disappointed by my not eating anything. So I had to explain, give reasons, sometimes even justify myself. This was no fun, and occasionally I would join in the eating 'out of politeness' or to avoid difficulties. At first I felt some aversion to eating, but subsequently I also quite enjoyed it. So I did on occasion take some food. However, the irregular cranking up of my digestive processes was uncomfortable, and I was always relieved when everything had settled down again afterwards.

After the 21-day process my weight had settled at 70 kilos. But about four months later I suddenly started to lose weight again for no apparent reason, although my energy level remained the same and I did not feel unwell. After taking advice I began to eat a small amount regularly, which enabled me to stabilize my weight, but I immediately began to lose again when I tried to stop eating once more. I didn't go into this strange phenomenon any more deeply because as things turned out I then decided to begin eating normally for a while. This was because my daughter, eleven years old at the time, had come to live with me. Considering her age and constitution I wasn't sure what effect it would have on her if her father always sat at the table but never ate with her.

I am very glad I undertook the 21-day process and would not want to have missed the experiences. I miss the condition of not eating, and now that I have started to eat regularly the positive changes I mentioned have receded: I get tired more quickly, need more sleep, and my varicose veins have returned. I frequently feel indisposed after eating because I experience my body as being overburdened. However, I no longer manage to do without food, for example when my daughter is away on a school trip or staying with friends. All in all I didn't find it too difficult to revert to eating at mealtimes once again since I know: 'The day eventually arrives when children leave home...!'

Benno Walbeck

Report by Sonja Hartmann

I am a mother of four children living in a small village on the border to Switzerland's central region. In addition to my household and work in the public health sector I was also following a part-time training as a class teacher in Waldorf education.

I came across the idea of living on light during the fifth semester of my studies and got hold of a copy of the book the following week. As I read I immediately felt the wish to experience the 21-day process. However, I realized that I would have to find within myself the strength to follow it through. So I trusted in the powers of the spirit and hoped that the right moment would turn up.

Nine months later I noticed that the small toe on my right foot was numb. And after a further two-and-a-half weeks I found myself in hospital having been diagnosed with a growth on the spinal marrow. I was virtually doubly incontinent and needed crutches to walk. I refused an operation which involved an 80% risk of ending up a paraplegic and I was also not willing to embark on chemotherapy. All I wanted was to go home.

While still in hospital I longed to meet someone who had experienced living on light. And while speaking to such a person I had the urgent feeling of already being in the midst of the process. Hence this diary.

Day 1, 1 a.m.
The food I ate at 8.30 yesterday evening is a great burden to my body, especially my legs, so much so that this is a further confirmation that I should open myself to something entirely new.

Day 3, 1 a.m.
I awoke with a start with a dry mouth and somewhat unstable circulation. Was able to pass water but I have not passed a motion since the first night. Writing has become important to me. A few hours ago I stepped out of the house on my crutches to get some fresh air. I implore God to give me a sign that following the 21-day process is the right way for me. I keep longing for God personally to give me encouragement during this time. 'Dear God, do not forget me!'

11 a.m.
After a bath with added organic vinegar, sour juice and sea salt, my mother made me a warm compress of equisetum on my back

which I hope will help. My mother is very good at giving gentle care.

1 p.m.
I look out of the window at the sky and watch the clouds as they change their shapes. Sometimes I think I see angels. From today I have begun to moisten my mouth with ice-cubes. It feels wonderful.

4 p.m.
I'm quite envious of my youngest daughter Jessica Irina having a snack on my lap: a bottle full of warm milk with chocolate powder.

10 p.m.
Propped on my crutches and accompanied by my mother I walk in the village for an hour. My dog comes too. I enjoy the night air.

Day 4, 3 a.m.
I wake up on command, as though forbidden to sleep any longer. It has been the same on previous nights. I go to the kitchen to rinse my mouth with ice-cubes. I enjoy the refreshing cold in my mouth and always take good care not to swallow any of the iced water. I am finding writing strenuous and my legs are wobbly. My body must have lost several kilos in weight. I'm thin. I don't want to lose my trust in God. I will believe that at least during this 21-day process I shall not die.

Day 5, 1 a.m.
I woke up after two hours sleep. I am quite aware that I don't look very attractive now. But I don't care! I'm surprised how wonderfully refreshing and cooling perfectly ordinary, tasteless

ice-cubes can be. My circulation is highly unstable. Can't risk going too far away from my bed.

2 a.m.

Although one is advised not to take a cold shower during these days I dared to have one anyway. It proved the right thing to do, since my body has been used to cold water all my life.

I am finding it really difficult to move on this fifth day. There's a rushing sound in my ears, I have circulation problems and a drawing pain in my back. On top of this I've started to menstruate unexpectedly. In the afternoon, with the help of my partner I go and lie down in the warm air beneath the big cherry tree behind the house to recover among natural surroundings. Towards evening I take a warm bath.

Day 6, 1 a.m.

Like a semi-desiccated flower crying out for water I lie for quite a while in the warm bath-water. It feels very good. Then I shower with cold water, which feels wonderful. Then I rinse my mouth with lemon water. An aroma of absolute freshness makes itself felt in my head.

5 a.m.

When I wake up I rinse my mouth alternately with water, lemon water and ice-cubes. I'm tremendously exited about the great day tomorrow. And, I'm still alive!

1 p.m.

I'm finding moving very difficult and am all the more grateful for the help my partner gives me. Thirst is getting increasingly demanding. My eyes are sunken, my cheeks hollow and my body emaciated. I have circulation problems, a drawing pain in my back, irregular menstruation, a rushing sound in my ears. When lying down my pulse is 64 but shoots up to 88 when I stand.

Day 7, midnight
I listen to my inner voice which says: 'Drink!' Until the eighth day I drink a decilitre every hour unless I fall asleep in between. At 1.15 a.m. by candlelight and in the company of my partner I ceremonially drink my first fruit juice with a teaspoon. It is very, very good! Every drop gives me a strong taste of orange in my mouth. I am happy.

11 a.m.
Every hour I very slowly sip a decilitre of fruit juice. In this careful way I hope to have accustomed my body to 'normal' drinking by midnight. I thank God often for his care of me, which I have felt during the course of these many days.

Day 8, 8.30 a.m.
Today I have already drunk a litre of liquid. My circulation is helping me feel stronger. My right leg feels very heavy and there is a strong tension in the lower calf. I thank God for his protection, which I sense.

6 p.m.
After another deep sleep, this time without any dream that I can remember, I fetch a glass of juice to my bedside in order gradually to gain some strength.

Day 9
I join other family members at the table at mealtimes. I'm drinking 5 litres of fruit juice a day. I find it such fun. From time to time I make a compress or lie in the bath to relax.

10 –11 p.m.
A night-time walk among green nature with my mother and my second-youngest child, together with the dog, is lovely.

Day 10, 6 p.m.
I am aware that I'm doing much more than the book says I should. I answer the phone, go to the doctor and get hold of all my files from the Canton hospital in order to arrange for my admission to the University Clinic in Zurich. I feel mentally loaded down by far too many things, much more so than I should. My mother helps me as best she can.

Day 12
In the middle of the day I spend a long time with my family in our beloved garden restaurant drinking 6 decilitres of mineral water and 2.5 of orange juice. Among the various fruit juices orange is my favourite. During the evening I worry about whether the process is still good for me with my body being so very thin. I go to sleep early and sleep through to the next morning.

Day 13, 8 a.m.
I feel light, and even my leg doesn't feel as heavy as it did in the past few days. But I keep having pins and needles in the second and third toe on my right foot.

11.30 a.m.
To detoxify my body I am still bathing with added salt, vinegar and juice every second day. My body is very, very thin. Since we don't have scales in the house I don't really know how much my weight has changed during the process so far. Should I be worried? Or if I knew, would I perhaps have lost the courage to continue with the process?

Day 14, 8 a.m.
I'm having muddled dreams. I also dream of eating. Motions are very small. It's a very beautiful day. I sleep a lot and drink a lot. For the first time in many days I want to try and cook lunch for the family. I enjoy it; of course without tasting the tiniest morsel! Towards evening I take a warm bath, as I have been doing over the past few days.

9.30 p.m.
Before going to bed I go for my night-time walk with my partner. My body feels light and I have hardly any discomfort.

Day 15, midnight
I'm lying awake in bed. More and more deeply I'm coming to realize how fundamentally important it is to live in the present moment. From now on I'm allowed to drink 40 per cent fruit juice. My body is getting stronger. I really enjoy cooking for the family. But I'm still worried about being so very thin.

Day 16
I receive an appointment for an examination at the University Clinic for 9 September. Bravo! If I'm still alive by then. I feel full of strength all day. I cook and bake a cake.

Day 18, 7 p.m.
Klaus brings scales home with him. He wants to be sure that my weight conforms with the book and is therefore remaining constant. I weigh 50.2 kilos.

Day 19, 7 a.m.
The scales show 49.7 kilos. The first visible signs of success show up today. I can stand on tip-toe again! And for the first time in three weeks I manage all day without crutches!

10.30 p.m.

After my bath I get into bed as usual with warm compresses. My weight is 50.9 kilos.

Day 20

I get up with a headache. Perhaps this is caused by the variety of fruit juices I've been drinking.

Day 21, 4 a.m.

With warm compresses on my tummy and back I watch a thunderstorm through the window from my bed. I used to be frightened of thunder and lightning. But now I feel so safe and protected that nothing in the world can be meaningless. I enjoy this moment.

10 p.m.

A warm bath, warm compresses and warm tea in bed. The scales show 50.4 kilos, just as the book says.

Day 22, 5.30 a.m.

The three weeks are over. I'm now free to do what I like with regard to eating. I cook and bake cake. My weight is now 49.6 kilos.

During the summer of 2004, 12 months after the first time, I went through the 21-day process again, this time, in comparison to the first, with much joy and no worries. My outer envelope and my inner self have never felt better! I feel that the tumour is still present in a small way. My next step — once again doing without normal nourishment — is planned for the spring of 2005.

Sonja Hartmann

Report by Angela-Sofia Bischof

Someone drew my attention to the article in *Das Goetheanum* which I had not noticed. The first time I read it I knew: This has been written for me! Having clarified the situation with my family I immediately took the decision to go ahead. The only possible time would begin two days later, and the whole process would have to be completed by five weeks later.

The process was to begin on Monday, 19 August 2002. My husband was prepared to give me the necessary support and peace. So I began my fast with much joy and enthusiasm in my own surroundings.

It was a very lovely time. Amid the radiant weather of high summer I was able to spend a great deal of time lying in our garden under the apple tree with its wonderful fragrance, watching the birds, the sky, the sun and all kinds of other things. I didn't feel hungry. Since I wasn't drinking anything my body seemed to get the message and was content. The wonderful fragrance of the apples soon taught me that communicating with our surroundings doesn't necessarily mean having to take a bite of the apple, just as you don't have to bite a person you love. Smelling, touching and enjoying the gifts of nature can also nourish us.

Of course I experienced some deterioration, but this was connected with the lack of fluids rather than of calories. (Dryness of the eyes should be treated with good eye-drops to avoid damaging them.) Of course you weaken during the first week. I lost 8 kilos, which naturally can't be regained overnight. But since I was able to lie down and could bath as often as I liked, external life was a challenge rather than a problem. In addition, glimpses of the other side of existence were so intense that the physical side receded more into the background.

I especially enjoyed the inner space which opened up at night.

All alone I was able to devote myself to my personal affairs and tasks and my own inner life's path. I needed little sleep and so was able to do what I liked with the remainder of the night. Even now I still need less sleep than I did before going through the process, so the time I have gained can be used for the purposes of 'inner hygiene'. I now stand more firmly on my feet and in the world than I would if I were to sleep the whole night away.

The first week, when you live entirely without liquids, was the most strenuous. You come very close to death, but you also receive the most precious gifts during that time. When you are so near the edge, many a gift tumbles 'over the fence' into your lap from the other side, and you can take these with you and use them when you rejoin other people.

I shall now describe the first week and its gifts.

During the first two days I was still under some stress concerning things that couldn't be put off until later. Towards the end of the second day I finally came to rest and was able to turn my attention to sorting out my own soul. The third day was one of peace and waiting. The fourth marked what was most important and — for me at least — most valuable, namely the beginning of the three days during which you undergo a process of being 're-modelled'. On each of these days you have to set aside three two-hour periods for this. For me this did not mean sleeping or just letting things happen but rather absolutely concentrated alertness and conscious attention to what was happening.

Above all else there was an exalted being of shining light and love who came to me with his helpers and worked on me with eager sincerity. I came to love him deeply, and after he had been to me a few times I asked whether he would be my friend. He consented, and we rejoiced together! I asked his name. It isn't easy to grasp a spiritual word that has no concept but only a sound, and reproduce it for human ears to hear. I thought it might be Alix, or Arix, but knew that this was not quite right. So when he came again I enquired once more. Again I couldn't really grasp it, but asked whether he would agree to my calling him 'Igor'. He did, and since then Igor has been my friend.

Apart from the periods when he was actually working on me, Igor also spent other times with me. He showed me the tasks he had to carry out in our earthly world. He is responsible for natural phenomena involving light, especially beautiful cloud formations lit up by the sun, sun-rises and sun-sets, rainbows and so on. All these things are generated in our world by spiritual beings. But they can only perceive them if we, in turn, are also aware of them and appreciate them in our soul, letting those beings experience them through us. So Igor and I showed each other the fruits of his work.

One morning when I was lying under my apple tree after an argument, Igor comforted me. He showed me the dewdrops in a special way. When I looked at the grass, all the dewdrops were blue. If I moved my head a tiny bit they were all green, or red, or orange – the grass was always adorned with jewels of the same colour. I had never seen dew in this way, but now I know how to do it. On another day, when there was a heavy shower while the sun still shone, he showed me elongated shining raindrops falling on the ground like liquid gold. These are images you never forget.

So I hardly had a chance to concern myself with bodily shortcomings. The world is so full of beauty which we hardly notice in the humdrum of daily life. This process of being close to death liberated me from everyday things and woke me up. In this way I passed the fourth, fifth and sixth days.

Keeping going with suitable awareness during the three fixed periods of being 're-modelled' each day was quite strenuous. The remaining time was hardly enough for bathing, reading and whatever else I wanted to do to carry on with my personal life, let alone rest. In my case some family decisions also needed to be discussed.

The seventh day is spent looking forward to drinking that first glass of liquid. I had decided on cranberry juice, diluted of course. This was not very suitable, but considering the character of the cranberry it was also very nice and valuable. The first sip after seven days of total abstinence was a thoroughly well-prepared 'sacred' event. During the following two weeks I drank mostly freshly-made apple juice from my tree, diluted with water.

After the first week I set out joyfully and with confidence on the path towards rebuilding my life and growing accustomed to it. But the rebuilding didn't seem to want to happen. I put on some weight but then lost it again. My strength didn't return and I felt dizzy. At first I tried some vegetable broth as a way of giving my body a little salt, but I didn't get any stronger and began to feel nervous. I contacted Michael Werner in the hope of profiting from his experience. But everyone's experience on this path is so different that although his help made me feel secure and calmed me down, my organism continued to react in its own way. After five weeks I capitulated and began to eat normally again. But I was determined to try the process again, next time in seclusion.

No sooner said than done! The time arrived four months later, on 17 November 2002. I was given the use of an apartment on the seventeenth floor of a block beside the Lake of Lucerne, an ideal situation for my project. I would even be allowed to use the block's internal sauna as often as I liked. The circumstances could not have been better.

This time I was much more active. The anxiety that is almost unavoidable on the first occasion did not reappear. I was sure I would succeed! I made use of what strength I had so long as I had it, and beyond, going out every day to walk along the lakeside, do some shopping or drive around the area. I used the sauna almost daily on a setting of gentle heat. Completely alone, hardly speaking with anyone, I devoted myself entirely to the process.

Once again I kept to the quiet periods from the fourth day onwards. But it became obvious that the 're-modelling' had been completed the first time round. So Igor mostly just sat by my bed and give me the gift of his company. Everything was noticeably more strenuous than the first time. Perhaps I exhausted myself too much with the sauna and the other activities. I got much more desiccated and my eyes suffered more. It took longer afterwards to build up to their accustomed freshness.

The sun shone and there was a strong foehn wind on the final day of the first week. I longed for water and drove down to the lake but couldn't find a spot where I might 'touch' the water and cool myself down. The foehn exhausted me and I kept having to stop for a rest, specially on the way back when I was walking into it and it played havoc with my dried-out eyes. Once back in the car on the way home I suddenly realized I didn't know the right way. I stopped at a petrol station and asked a man who was filling his car. He looked at me and was visibly shocked – I really did look as though I was at death's door. He got out his map and showed me the way, and as I left he said to me: God bless you! That man's words moved me in the depths of my soul. They flowed into me like a healing balm, giving me warmth, comfort and strength. The love of a human brother had touched me, and as I drove on my eyes filled with tears.

That, then, was the first, difficult week of my second attempt to convert to a way of receiving nourishment through the soul. Once again there was the sacred act of the first draught. My body absorbed the liquid and I began to put on weight. But soon I experienced and then accepted that my body did not want this. The 21 days were nearly over and again I grew nervous as my weight decreased. I was of course sad and at a loss, so I decided to ask for advice and an answer from 'the other side'. And I was not let down: The process which I had twice gone through — unsuccessfully — gave me the opportunity to experience for myself what I had been guilty of doing to others long, long ago. It was an ancient karmic debt about which I was already aware. To live without food is not my task, but rather to be conscious of what I do with it. This was the answer, plain and clear.

So what was now left for me, apart from the very valuable experience I had gained? The most important thing is my friendship with Igor. This again and again breaks through to my consciousness in the many and varied beauties of the world around me, but it is also ever-present in the fundamental understanding of myself that lives in my soul. Then there is the extra 'free time' already mentioned because I still need less sleep than before, and also my much more conscious attitude to food and the gifts of nature — whereby I constantly realize that it is actually not necessary to take these gifts into yourself if you have practised and learned to nourish the body by means of a loving awareness. Reverence, earnestness and gratitude come to be like the river bed along which the power of nature's gifts can flow into your body.

The path described above and the experiences gained along the way are founded, 'earthed', in a biography that followed an entirely ordinary course. I have been married for 43 years, had four children, and always enjoyed enough time and space in which I could follow my own inner path. When I began the process for the first time I was 61 years old.

Angela-Sofia Bischof

Report by Günther Becker

I was born in 1926 and am the father of two sons. My wife died in 1986. I worked as an electrical engineer in the field of electronic control technology for 30 years. I've been a pensioner since 1988, and since 1994 have been living in a farmhouse on about a hectare of land with fruit trees, first with one of my sons, but for the last few years alone. So, entirely in the positive sense, there is 'nothing to disturb me'. I do sport, cross-country skiing — in 2005 I took part for the sixteenth time in the Engadine ski marathon — and javelin throwing.

In August 2002 I was in the midst of the fruit harvest when I suddenly began to feel fed up with all the bother of gathering food, cooking and the other jobs involved. I then came across Michael Werner's article 'Not by bread alone', which had just appeared. After reading the very first sentences I knew: 'Living on light! That's it!' I read the article several times with increasing enthusiasm, and soon decided: 'I am going to try that!' So I straight away got hold of the book *Living on Light* by Jasmuheen and immersed myself in the instructions about the 21-day process. And a few weeks later I began to follow that path. Living on my own, with 'nothing to disturb me', I was able to remain in my own home.

How was it possible for me to reach a decision so quickly? Looking back on my life up to that point, I think two personal experiences and developments helped: Firstly I had frequently concerned myself with many different aspects of food and eating, and secondly I had always striven to make what was good within me more effective.

In brief: From 1950 onwards my parents and I became vegetarians and chose the Waerland Method, a lacto-vegetable diet which I continued with my wife after our marriage in 1960. In the late 1960s, in order to take account of our children's social relationships with their friends, we began to eat more cooked food. For quite a while in the early 1990s I ate exclusively raw produce in the hope of curing my chronic sinusitis. However, I only succeeded in this in 1993 after applying Johann Gander's method of enlivening the forces in water, which made me aware of the importance of water quality. From then to 2002 I ate cooked food according to the principle which uses the different cereals in rhythmic combination with the seven days of the week. As to mental effort, I worked with yoga as well as physical and breathing exercises during the 1960s and 70s, in the hope of improving my thinking capacities. I have been interested in anthroposophy since 1976 and also general knowledge about the human being through the lectures given by Berthold Wulf.

Even when I was young I was sure that receiving nourishment from light could be possible, being impressed by the examples of Nicholas von der Flüe and Therese of Konnersreuth and reports about monks and hermits surviving on extremely little food. Later I heard of other interesting examples from the Indian region. In Unerhörtes aus der Medizin by Jürg Reinhard and Adolf Baumann I found indications about being nourished through breathing and via the sense organs. As time went on, all this must have prepared me for being able to make up my mind so rapidly to take up living on light in August 2002.

The 21-day process ran without anything special happening. The most noticeable effect in the early days was a change in the oral cavity. My mouth felt and looked as though it was on fire; everything was bright red. By consulting a health dictionary I was able to reassure myself that it wasn't scarlet fever. I cooled my tongue and oral mucus with chunks of ice, spitting out the resulting water in order to keep to the rule of the 21-day process not to take in any fluids. I felt quite weak during the process, but there was no need for me to exert myself during that time.

During the early weeks after completing the process I felt very well, and I also discovered that I had more strength in my arms even though they were now thinner. For some days I had a sense that my body was internally invulnerable to attack through illness and that nothing could gain a foothold within it. After a few weeks the sensation of heat in my mouth was also milder, although it was still present and still made me want to cool it down. Mindful of the basic premise 'Drinking yes, eating no' I reasoned that ice-cream was really nothing but frozen fluid which I could therefore imbibe. At first I took care to choose low-calorie varieties since I didn't want to cheat and eat food after all. But after some time I began taking other varieties which tasted better, but always only in small amounts. Then I began to take a little chocolate as well, and now I've arrived at sucking 'sweets', i.e. the only thing I still crave is the sweetness of sugar.

What is my situation today? The desire to have something in my mouth is strongest when I'm nervous, for example if I find myself running out of time with a project I'm trying to finish; and afterwards, when I'm able to relax, or doing something passive like watching television. The desire recedes most when I'm thinking hard, concentrating on something or meditating, learning a poem by heart, or paying attention to something new that interests me; also during physical activity such as chopping wood or throwing the javelin.

Based on the above realizations, my aim now is to reach the stage of being entirely nourished by light alone, but without wanting to force this by feeling that I am being influenced by powers 'from above'.

Günther Becker

Report by Catherine Zimmermann

It all began seven years ago. After a big disappointment and a small operation performed under anaesthetic I found myself thrown back on my own devices and entirely alone in my apartment. In tears I called out: 'God, take me with you!' For the first time in my life I would have been perfectly happy to die. But of course I also knew very well that escape is not so simple and that life was really only just beginning. I resolved to change my life from its very foundations.

For seven years I lived only on raw foods, fruit and raw vegetables such as carrots, salad, herbs, fennel and so on; also nuts and almonds. For a year and a half I only ate fruit. Occasional backache, bladder infections, acne, pain in the kidneys and menstrual discomfort, and even the beginnings of cellulitis, all disappeared entirely.

I have always known intuitively that it must be possible to live without eating anything at all. I attended yoga classes and did body-awareness exercises, later eurythmy, circle dance and initiation dance. Whenever I did a lot of exercises or spent much time in the open air I managed on really small amounts of food, but I didn't have the courage to take this further. At Christmas 2003 I heard about the possibility of being nourished by light and about a certain Dr Michael Werner, whom I then contacted. I bought Jasmuheen's book *Living on Light*. And early in 2004 I followed the 'process' in accordance with the book's instructions.

What I remember most was having a lot of time, which I really enjoyed. Everything was so quiet and peaceful! It was very beneficial. I could spend hours washing myself, chewing snow and spitting it out, lighting my wood-burning stove, observing nature and lovingly paying attention to myself. There was no 'must', so I rested, prayed, dozed, slept, hoped ... I was happy. Bumping my head on a sloping rafter released a flood of tears;

for the first time in ages I had a really good cry. Everything took a long time and much effort. Sometimes I groaned like an old woman, and my head ached. I imagined how lovely it would be to drink again and longed for the fine fruits in the market. During the first week I mostly felt very hot. When I went for a walk my step was so light. Later I heard a woman say about me that she had 'seen something shining walking up the path'. Sometimes, more in the second and third week, I played my flute, did yoga and eurythmy, read the Bible, wrote my diary, drew pictures and modelled with clay. I did not use any electricity but had candlelight and fragrant oil burners.

On Wednesday, 10 March 2004, the eleventh day of the process, I wrote in my diary:

'How quickly the days are passing. Today I slept as much as I needed. As to the way I pass the day, I let myself be led entirely by my "inner guide". I even went on the swing for a bit, and had a look at the tree-house. Wrapped in my layers of woollies, moving about made me feel warm. It is wonderful to be so quiet. Even when I do jobs I go entirely at my own pace. Sometimes I talk loudly, yet it's so quiet ... I enjoy being allowed to see the crocuses and daffodil buds, the sprouting green and the sun. Who knows what the weather is going to do. How strange to see the palm fronds covered in snow. Will I feel like chewing snow again? Or drinking it? Perhaps it will give me strength, since it is adapted to the climate. Now I'm lovely and warm. It feels good. I might try and describe my condition as follows: I feel that I'm being left alone, protected, loved, respected, at peace. I can only partially feel my body, in the places where there's still some "illness". Like something in my throat ... Well, actually I can feel my body if I concentrate.'

After the 21-day process I didn't find it easy to move back to town, but I managed fairly well. I weighed only 45 kilos (my height being 1.63 m). I left the cabin with my heavy rucksack and the first person I met was the bus driver. I went back to work and for a while still kept going on the diluted fruit juice I had been drinking during the second and third weeks of the process. Things went quite well. Then one morning I fainted and came to myself with a big bruise on my head. I was disappointed, and changed over to home-pressed pure fruit juices. And soon I was also eating fruit, which seems more practical and suits me better. Although I had a lot of work, I remained 'stable' over the summer eating large amounts of fruit (fresh figs, tomatoes, melons) and swimming in the lake, all while weighing 50 to 52 kilos.

From the days when I ate only raw vegetables I'm used to people giving me funny looks on occasion, and I don't mind so much any more. Sometimes I make people curious, sometimes I irritate them. Some find me irresponsible (lack of vitamins, protein, enzymes) and others think I'm crazy. My parents and brother have accepted the way I live as regards food. Of course it's fun to eat with others, but there are also other things you can do together, like hiking, dancing, making music ... The most important thing is that everyone is healthy and contented!

I soon noticed that there were many foods I no longer fancied, and I can easily do without these. So at present my diet consists of fruit only. This seems to me to be the only 'physical' form of nourishment that is entirely complete in itself and self-contained. One piece of fruit left as nature made it is a blessing. I find combining different foods intrusive and a compromise.

Light – everything is contained within it.

Catherine Zimmermann

Report by Ingrid Axenbeck

My deeply-felt wish and search for a way of life that could combine spirituality with everyday life led me to embark on the process of being nourished by light in 1999. Prior to that I had repeatedly become bogged down in everyday matters, and I was also in the midst of a difficult life situation. As a teacher at a state school, I wanted to begin the 21-day process during the long summer holiday. I asked my second son to look after the house, the dog and two cats. Then, on 17 August 1999, after two days on a detox fast, I withdrew to my room.

The process ran very harmoniously and it was a profound spiritual experience. I am now finding that it marked the beginning of a wonderful journey which is still on-going. Unlike those around me, I did not find it a problem to entrust my physical existence to the care of others. In addition, I am now able to recognize and resolve patterns of belief and blockages. Being able to use the 'violet flame' as a marvellous tool is a wonderful gift from the spiritual world. I am filled with gratitude and love in being led more and more to understand my own divine origins and recognize Christ within me.

As an aside I would like to mention a 'coincidence': I have since realized that I was just seven times seven years old when I began the process. The first seven days ended on 23 August, my forty-ninth birthday. I feel newly born.

Ingrid Axenbeck

Report by Wiltrud Schmidt

In the summer of 2002 the journal *Das Goetheanum* carried an interview on the subject of receiving nourishment from light. A. 52-year-old man with increasing health problems and a tendency to be overweight talked about his decision to undertake the 21-day process that opens up the possibility of being nourished by light without the need for any solid food.

I had never heard of people in Central Europe being able to function in an ordinary job and cope with all that entails as well as other professional and personal commitments – in short, being able to lead an active life – without physical food. Of course I had come across instances of individuals who lived an intensely meditative or religious life in solitude far from any active work commitments while surviving without solid food, and indeed in some cases without any fluids either, such as Nicholas von der Flüe or Therese of Konnersreuth. But surely this was a different matter. As I read the article I began to realize that as someone born in the final years of the Second World War who had known what it felt like to be hungry I had become a person who enjoyed eating, especially eating good food, and who possessed 'the stomach of a horse'. So I decided that 'not eating' was emphatically not for me. I could imagine, however, that in this age of increasing individualism there might be some who could follow that path, but I was not one of them. So I thought in the year 2002.

Since I had always had very little spare time away from my professional commitments, I had quite early on adopted the strategy of concentrating on a single theme for several months at a time without being tempted to read several books on different subjects all at once, which would only have exacerbated the lack of coherence I experienced in my daily work. I had made a conscious decision not to be tempted. I was thus familiar with the idea of exercising the will even though I did so without any knowledge of a spiritual background or reason. But I was used to making a decision and then using my will to carry it through and bring it to a conclusion. For many years I was also accustomed to fasting during Easter Week.

When I discovered anthroposophy in 1980 my whole life gained a new foundation. At last I was able to integrate the various parts of it with the help of a view of the world that gave me a sense of direction. Over the years, this orientation had influenced the capacities and strengths I possessed, gradually transforming them. Some had disappeared from one part of me and reappeared in another. In my youth I had been involved in a lot of sport and been physically very active. This had made me physically agile, strong and persevering; will forces were schooled at that level which, having undergone a transformation, could later be applied to new tasks. These processes of transformation had often caused external physical changes which always signalled that something 'was going on' in my body, for example in my breathing, my circulation, or my joints. Such phenomena were familiar to me and I experienced them in various ways. I knew that all the symptoms were a consequence of the path of schooling and were therefore necessary, since only then could a metamorphosis come about. So even though they might be uncomfortable, incapacitating or painful, I had to recognize them for what they were, accept them and support the process that was under way. It would not have been good, on the other hand, to block or prevent them, for example by following some well-meaning medical advice.

Having begun in the spring of 2004, some processes of this kind were once again reaching a climax. Impressive images I experienced one weekend for the first time brought about changes in my diet. This was entirely new to me. For weeks I ate nothing but bread and honey: honey for breakfast, honey for lunch, and again honey in the evening. My craving for the honey-pot was almost greedy, and yet I had no need for any other kind of food. This phase ended quite suddenly, and I had no idea why. It was replaced by a similar period of craving for meat. I was experiencing needs and changes in diet which I had never known before; and the healthy appetite I had enjoyed all my life was also waning gradually. All this went on inside me without my knowing the reason or being able to influence the changes in any way. There was no conscious decision of will. But I also felt entirely confident that everything was alright even though I had no idea why. I continued with my meditative life as usual.

In July 2004 a complete reversal of my digestive function and food requirement then came into play within the space of 24 hours: I experienced a clear and distinct need to stop eating solid food. Although I was still to some extent under the sway of modern medicine, which dictates that human beings need fats, carbohydrates, proteins, vitamins and many other substances in order to live, I knew, thanks to that article, that there are some people to whom this doesn't apply. Yet it still took some effort before I could accept that I was now one of those people. The needs of my body, however, were so clear and unequivocal that I was able to come to terms with it all.

For breakfast I now have a fruit tea, and for lunch and supper I drink delicious fruit or vegetable juices, or in winter some hot vegetable broth.

I have informed my friends and acquaintances about the changes that have come about in me, adding that I have no fixed idea or specific motive in mind and saying that if tomorrow I were to feel the need to eat again I would certainly do just that. I still go out for meals with them, and as I sit there with my glass of tomato juice in front of me I apologize to the waiter for not ordering anything else. My friends enjoy their meal and I enjoy watching them enjoying themselves. I experience the sight of the food on their plates very intensely, and also the smells. But that is quite enough. I don't feel hungry and neither do I have any desire to eat some of it. The best part for me has been that all my friends have tolerated my needs; instead of trying to persuade me otherwise, they have accepted that I can take responsibility for myself. One or another may have found it none too easy, but when we 'eat' together everything goes quite smoothly.

As before, I am beginning to notice a change. My ability to concentrate has grown, I become aware of things at the right moment, my common sense is more wide awake and I am stronger at being able to act in accordance with it. My thought life is more alive and imaginative. There are also some uncomfortable consequences. For example I easily feel cold, and my legs tend to swell. But these situations are temporary, they are bearable, and one day they will either disappear or I will learn to handle them. So life is full of surprises that call for presence of mind and mental agility to accompany this balancing act between willpower and the ability to adjust.

In an essay written in 1927 Ita Wegman mentioned Therese of Konnersreuth in connection with the anthroposophical view of doing without food in the twentieth century.* She regarded such a thing as being pathological at that time for people who needed to carry out tasks in the world, but she added that a time would come in human evolution when it would be possible to manage without food. In view of the increasing impurity, contamination and pathogenic alteration in foodstuffs in our time, all of which are likely to increase further, it is quite possible to imagine that in the not too distant future the fruits of the earth will no longer guarantee healthy nourishment for human beings.

So abstention from food, for whatever reason, on the one hand, and the decreasing quality of food on the other, could be two phenomena which both point in the same direction. We shall have to wait and see how the need for nourishment will develop in every individual in future times.

Wiltrud Schmidt

---

*Wegman, 1927.

Report by Clio Osman

I was born in Oregon, USA, in June 1941. Even as a young child I was always asking: Where have I come from, why am I here, where am I going? This led to my being baptized in the Catholic church at the age of 12. Later I became a nun. I had always been fascinated by the saints, and I had already heard extraordinary accounts of people who lived 'on light alone'. After seven years as a nun during which time I also trained as a teacher, my path led me on to teaching in ghettos near San Francisco, the Peace Corps in the Philippines, and travel in Asia. This ended in Britain where I discovered Emerson College – the Rudolf Steiner teacher-training college – 'by accident' and recognized anthroposophy as my true path through life. I studied eurythmy and then worked first in Britain and later at a Waldorf school in southern Germany.

As I have mentioned, I had known about the phenomenon of living on light for a long time without realizing that this is also possible for 'ordinary mortals'. At some point I heard about people, mainly in Australia, who were nourished by light. I thought this absurd at the time and immediately forgot all about it. But when I saw an announcement about Michael Werner's lecture in Stuttgart I was curious, and went. He had hardly finished his first sentence when I knew: I'm going to do this.

Other reasons gradually contributed to my decision. I think that spiritual work is easier to do when you are living on light because your physical organism isn't burdened by digestive processes and suchlike, and because the 'food' you are ingesting is pure. Many people had reported that they needed less sleep, and I had been suffering from tiredness for years. As a person living alone I would also save time through not having to cook or do much shopping. And it would be nice to have the money to spend on other things. But the most important reason for me was that one would be living proof of the fact that there are other things besides materialism in our world. This was a particular concern of mine, especially as my family were extremely materialistic in their outlook.

Initially I wanted to go through the process during the summer holidays, but seeming obstacles kept interfering. I was fortunate in finding someone willing to stand by me for the whole time provided that I had a medical doctor willing to be available at all times. Since my own doctor regarded the whole thing as total nonsense, I asked an anthroposophical practitioner whether he would be available for the planned period. I told only my closest female friends about my plan, and they were not best pleased. On a visit to Michael Werner who set aside several hours for us, my accompanying friend and I received satisfactory answers to all our questions. He also offered to accompany me during the process and made himself available by telephone for almost the whole of the 21 days.

I carried out the process in my own home, exactly following the instructions in Jasmuheen's book *Living on Light*. I was absolutely sure that everything would run smoothly so long as I kept to the instructions. I also knew that I could break off at any time if things should not go well. I informed my friends that I would not be available for the period in question because I intended to follow a kind of 'retreat'. I had bought a large air mattress for my living room as an extra resting place (the process stipulates a great deal of bed rest). About two years earlier I had also begun regular fitness workouts, which had made me more mobile (I have arthritis) and improved my weight. For the weeks leading up to the beginning of the process I had also switched over to a diet that didn't place too much strain on the digestive system. So then my journey began.

Since I had decided not to keep a diary, the following is what I can still recall after an interval of almost a year. We began the process joyously with a modest celebration. I slept well and spent the first two days reading an exciting novel. Real thirst did not arise until the third day. My friend had bought small plastic containers for making ice-cubes, so I was able to suck these with increasing frequency and thus soothe the dryness of my mouth. The greatest problem at that moment were strong muscular pains in my buttocks caused by having sat for two long in one position while reading. Even on my waterbed the pain was such that I could hardly sleep. I waited eagerly for the events described by Jasmuheen but noticed nothing that resembled becoming attached to a 'spiritual drip'. Although I grew noticeably weaker during the following days we took a daily walk which always did me good. I also had a strong need for coldness, and as there was snow on the ground outside my door I frequently went out to rub my hands and also my face vigorously with snow.

My companion found it remarkable that despite the process my face continued to look so well. Of course I lost weight, but I was convinced that this would settle down in due course. Apart from the pains already mentioned I had no particular physical problems. Even on the seventh day we went for our walk, but I did need to keep stopping for a breather. My urge to drink became almost unbearable, so I decided to take the first sip on the evening of the seventh day at around 8 p.m. Once again we combined this with a small ceremony. Whether or not it was too soon for that drink I don't know, but in my experience drinking was not as wonderful as I had expected. In fact, after the second sip I even vomited.

Then I entered a very peculiar state. I had arrived in a kind of 'intermediate space' where my sense of place and time was unreal and displaced into a kind of dream existence. I had the illusion of having to drink for two persons, and the nightmare persisted almost throughout the night during which I sweated profusely. When I woke up the peculiar state was gone. Although I still needed a great deal of rest, the physical building-up phase had begun which I expected would lead to a gradual gain in weight. Since this did not happen in the days that followed I became anxious, but Herr Werner kept assuring me that everything was alright. In keeping with the division of the process into three seven-day periods I noticed that now, in the second week, I was no longer so concerned with physical cleansing but rather with matters of the soul. I thought about many things and reached some enlightening conclusions regarding my feelings. In the middle of that week I also had an irresistible urge to 'tidy up', so there followed a huge clearing out project that lasted for two days. I grew stronger daily and drank a great deal, as Herr Werner had suggested. At the beginning of the third week I sensed that now it was time to tackle my spiritual life. It was wonderful to have so much peace, to be alone with myself without any interruptions, and to read.

At the end of the 21-day process I had one day before school began. I was slightly worried because I wasn't sure how many people knew I had been doing the process and how they would react. In the event, only one teacher mentioned it, and I thought I noticed some of the children looking askance at me. I was still somewhat weak, but was able to sit down during my lessons. My thoughts and feelings were very clear during that period, and this enabled me to master my days with ease.

But then a problem arose which I had not foreseen. My office was situated right next to the school kitchen so that I was always able to smell what was for lunch. This bothered me, and so did thoughts of tasting 'something delicious'. I stuck to my guns at first because I really wanted to persevere, since that would be the only way 'to make it all worthwhile'. But as time went on I began to chew a few morsels and then spit them out although I didn't feel at all good doing this. Then I began to drink broth regularly. Healthwise I felt very well even though I still wasn't putting on any weight, which worried me. A friend, a medical doctor who visited me at the time said later that she was not sure whether I had indeed successfully completed the process since I seemed to her to be so open and unprotected. A few weeks later I began to pass regular motions whereupon I rapidly lost weight. Since I also began to look ill I knew that – for whatever reason – I must begin to eat again. I had no difficulty in doing so.

I asked friends who possess the ability to perceive spiritually whether I had really succeeded with the process. Their reply was 'Yes and No'. And when I asked when I could continue with living on light the answer I received was: 'In ten years time.' Looking back I am glad to have had the experience but not sad about having ceased to live in that way. We shall see whether I do begin again.

Clio H. Osman

Report by Peter Zollinger

I was born in 1952, married in 1974 and have two adult sons. By profession I'm an entrepreneur.

About seven years ago my neighbour handed Jasmuheen's book on the phenomenon of being nourished by light over the garden fence to me. 'You've got to read this,' she said, 'it's extremely interesting.' I took it partly out of interest and partly so as not to offend my neighbour.

At the time I was going through a phase of reading a lot of so-called 'positive' books, and those close to me had slowly grown accustomed to the fact that my ideas about life, death and our task on the earth differed from those we are taught in school.

The phenomenon of living on light fascinated me so much once I had read the book that I immediately thought I would like to feed myself in this way. So I told my family. But this was just too far removed from normality for my nearest and dearest. After her initial bafflement my wife went quiet. That evening she cooked my favourite dish, but instead of food she placed three tea-lights on my plate. I can still picture the scene: three plates of lasagne and one of light for the main course. We all laughed heartily, and my wife had successfully cured me of my illusion of living on light, for at that time this was indeed merely a wish and not yet a goal.

Seven years later, in May 2004, I came across a report by someone who was practising this 'miracle' in Switzerland. This time I really wanted to know about it, so I arranged to meet Herr Werner who was the subject of the report. I intended to collect facts as a basis for whatever decision I might make. Our conversation was very objective and open in every respect and Herr Werner appeared to be a completely 'normal' person. Apart from his somewhat ill-fitting trousers there was nothing at all unusual about the man, and certainly nothing that pointed to his rather remarkable talent. The modesty of his behaviour was for me the main reason for trusting what he had to say and so the path he had decided to tread came to seem worthy of imitation.

Having convinced myself that I had found an effective way of maintaining my physical health while promoting my inner life I began to prepare those around me for the coming change. Resistance, especially from those closest to me, was massive, only this time my wish had become one hundred per cent intention and I was therefore no longer prepared to be so easily influenced by them. I had reflected thoroughly on Charmaine Harley's questionnaire; in other words I had made myself aware of any subliminal doubts I might have had and sorted them out.

Without the conviction that arose out of this awareness-raising exercise I would not have overcome the hurdles I encountered before and during the 21-day process as easily as I did. With hindsight, after successfully completing the process but subsequently failing to pursue that way of life permanently, I have asked myself what the true reason for my decision could have been. I have come to realize that in addition to the aspects of health, time-saving and increased efficiency, the main reason was to raise myself to a higher wave-length in order to cope better with the tasks I was facing in life.

At the end of June 2004 I rented an apartment attached to a friend's house in the same village for 21 days and told my wife that I would not be contacting anyone for three weeks, that no one except my son who worked in our family firm should visit me and that no one else was even to know where I was.

My son accompanied me throughout the whole process in a very loving way, even though he couldn't understand my decision. He said: 'You are my father, and you have good reasons for what you think and do; I accept that, even though I don't understand it.' He visited me almost daily except when he was too far away. I had asked him not to mention anything to do with our family business during the three weeks, and he kept to this strictly. Together with Michael Werner, whom I was allowed to contact regularly by telephone, my son was a great help, especially when I suddenly got the hiccups after three days which continued to bother me for the next four. After four days of the hiccups every contraction of my diaphragm was so painful that I could have screamed; and this lengthy attack had also weakened me further. Fortunately I had worked out a very full programme of activities with almost no empty moments. So the pain was not as troublesome during the day as it was at night, when I sometimes lay curled up and awake for hours on end. This sounds dreadful, but actually it was this very pain that taught me how to recognize a situation I did not like for what it was and accept it without protesting. This capability gave me strength, and suddenly the pain became only a fraction of what it had been while I was trying to fight it. Today I am grateful for that 'torture'. Thanks to my good schedule I was never bored for a moment during the process. There was always something to do: write a letter, read a book – for example the Bible, a biography of the Dalai Lama, a thriller – make plans for the future, write down an analysis of the process, go for a walk, enjoy planned rest periods, listen to classical music, try to understand myself, find contact with the sphere of causality, gain answers to my questions through clear images, and much else.

The three weeks flew by, and I remember them as one of the most enjoyable times in my life. After completing the process I remained physically weak, and on the occasion of a birthday party with a gigantic buffet I allowed myself to be tempted to eat. Now, three months later, I am still eating regularly. But in spite of this I recommend the 21-day process to anyone who is seriously striving to live more consciously. From the process itself as well as my subsequent relapse I have gained important insights which are helping me tackle life with a lighter touch even though I am not living on light. At the very least I have taken a step forward in humility. As a result I have become more relaxed and at the same time more courageous. I consciously acknowledge my bodily systems for the efforts they make on my behalf.

Of course I would still hope to learn how to absorb energy from the cosmos, but in the final analysis I am no longer all that concerned as to whether I shall ever live exclusively 'on light'. I now feel it is much more important to begin facing up to problems rather than avoiding tasks by 'skating over them or rising above them'. It was this tendency to flee that had lain hidden behind my grand reasons for embarking on the 21-day process. I have also come to realize that attaining either a physical or a spiritual goal releases energy which only enhances one's awareness if one has decided in advance what actual purpose it is to serve. In other words, in future I shall put the energy that results from achieving an aim towards an additional effort for which I would lack the strength if I had failed to achieve that aim. Or in other words: I can achieve more because I reach more goals. This only became clear to me in consequence of my efforts to throw light on my relapse. From this point of view, my failure to live exclusively 'on light' could even be seen as a greater blessing than success would have been, and this insight is now giving me the strength to strive for a conscious solution to my present tasks and problems.

Peter Zollinger

Report by Gertrud Müller

I live at Minusio beside Lake Maggiore. Walking down along the Navegna, a torrent that rushes over impressive granite boulders, I can reach the lake in five minutes and there enjoy its beauty together with the wooded slopes and picturesque villages on the other shore.

I am a retired home economics teacher, unmarried, living alone and comfortably off. Having taught for many years, including 13 at the Ittigen Rudolf Steiner School, and having then spent two-and-a-half years helping establish the kitchen at the new old people's home at Rüttihubelbad, I finally taught gardening and worked as a member of the college of teachers at the Locarno Rudolf Steiner School for a reduced number of hours until my seventieth birthday. I'm now enjoying my freedom in my small garden and beautifully situated apartment in

the Canton of Ticino. I have joined reading groups and participate in eurythmy and folk dance classes. Meditation and prayer
as well as short eurythmy exercises and playing the flute are all
included in my daily routine. I enjoy cooking (vegan) and do my
own cleaning in addition to caring for two garden plots by the
side of the flats. I feel very secure and at home here in southern
Switzerland.

When I read Thomas Stöckli's interview with Dr Werner I
immediately felt attracted to the impulse of living on light and
could not stop thinking about it. That was on 20 August 2002.
After studying Jasmuheen's book *Living on Light* I decided to
embark on the process on 13 September. I was hoping that my
general health would improve. I also thought the experience
would be very valuable in showing people going hungry all over
the world, especially in southern parts of the globe, that it is
possible to live on light rather than on food, something which is
already practised a good deal by those leading a spiritual life in
Africa and Asia.

I gave away all the food I had in the house, keeping only the
fruit juices I would be needing. I found a dear and capable friend
here in Ticino who was prepared to visit me once a day during
this interesting period and accompany me in her thoughts.

I took Charmaine Harley's self-screening questionnaire very
seriously and endeavoured to feel in harmony with the sacred-
ness of the process. I have adhered to the vegan diet for many
years and enjoy eating very much which, however, has become
more questionable now that genetic engineering has been
brought to bear on the food question. Right from the beginning,
being someone who loves moving about and working, I did not
take the need for withdrawing from everything 'worldly'
seriously enough. I took two short walks to the lake every day
and continued to enjoy working in my small garden and caring

for the flowers on two balconies as well as my indoor plants. And on the eighth day I even attended a wonderful orchestral concert at Locarno with a friend. Subsequently I experienced this as being unacceptable to the spirits accompanying me. They only gave me back their support after I had felt profound remorse and sincerely implored them to forgive me. This shook me up a good deal.

By being too active during the process I broke the rules, and so I lost too much weight, having already been quite thin at the outset. But I still felt very well at the end of the three weeks, even though somewhat weak. And looking back I realize that I was again too eager to get going and be active.

Regarding my experiences during the process I can say that I felt very well on my first day without breakfast and went happily to work energetically in my garden (which, as I have said, I should not have done). I also experienced my short walks to the lake in a new way. These walks helped me breathe deeply, and led me to sit on a granite boulder warmed by the sun to admire the sparkling water while I absorbed nourishment from the light. I then used to rest on my balconies which faced either the morning or the afternoon sun and enjoy the peace, the rushing of the stream and all of nature in a new way. On the evening of the third day I was tempted to bathe in the warm lake, which I enjoyed. Before going to sleep I tuned in to the departure of my 'spiritual body'. One night I dreamt of a golden shaft of light running right through me. It was a vertical shaft, but I couldn't tell whether it was coming down to me or rising up from me. But it was a spiritual experience which impressed me greatly. Afterwards I felt that the golden shaft had come down to me and filled me with wonderful strength. After that I discovered a verse by Rudolf Steiner which begins as follows:

May God's protective ray of blessing
Fill my growing soul,
That it may take hold of
Strengthening forces everywhere...

This verse has since then accompanied me on my journey into each new day. It reminds me of that wonderful feeling of being pierced through by the golden shaft from heaven.

After the third day I was preoccupied by my dry mouth, and I was glad to be able to rinse it and suck ice-cubes more or less frequently and then spit out the water. Apart from this I felt well and enjoyed the lovely autumn weather, resting at regular intervals, reading and sleeping, and going for those forbidden short walks to the lake. As I awoke after the mid-day sleep on the fourth or fifth day I sensed a figure of light hovering beside and above me. I felt as though it were aiming a small watering can at my back, the etheric 'drip' which, as I later read in the book *Living on Light*, might be inserted near the kidneys. Going over this experience again later I found it a wonderful, tender, loving gesture which allowed me to perceive with amazement and gratitude the work of the heavenly brotherhood and the spiritual beings which strengthened me greatly.

Towards evening on the seventh day one is allowed to drink for the first time. I relished the first longed-for sip of water with deep gratitude as a wonderful gift from God. It was like an invigorating blessing deep down in my human nature. And I felt the same when I solemnly and festively took the first fruit juice.

Jasmuheen's instructions for the eighth to the twenty-first day accompanied me throughout that phase. I re-read the biography of Nicholas von der Flüe with deeper understanding, and also Jesus Christ's conversation with the Samaritan woman beside Jacob's well and his subsequent conversation with his disciples

(John 4). It was at this time that I met an architect from Sarnen who often visits the hermitage of Nicholas von der Flüe beside the Ranft. After completing the process I visited the hermitage for the first time. On that cold and rainy afternoon in the company of my tactful and sensitive companion I was deeply moved by experiencing this special location with a subtle and newly-awakened spiritual sensitivity. Afterwards I felt very weak and thoroughly chilled and yet also enriched in a wonderful way.

Throughout the process I was able to telephone Herr Werner for advice if I had questions or felt uncertain. I greatly appreciated this and he gave me valuable help. On 3 October, two days after completing the process, I participated in the communion service of the Christian Community. I had a far more profound experience than usual, and the Host was my first bite of solid food. I allowed it to melt slowly in my mouth and thoughtfully 'incorporated' it into my body together with the freshly-pressed biodynamic grape juice: an entirely new experience of profoundly-felt gratitude for 'food and drink'.

In the days that followed I drank juice at mealtimes and felt well. A trip to the Swiss National Exhibition Centre two weeks later took me to the limit of my strength, and I found it difficult not to eat anything. Then I went to visit my friends in Palermo, which I have been doing several times a year for a long time. They were only willing to have me as a guest if I promised to eat; otherwise I would have to find somewhere else to stay. I didn't want to go ahead and lose this intimate closeness with my friends, especially as I was due to fly to Colombo, Singapore and Melbourne immediately afterwards. I no longer needed any medication after completing the process and took none with me on my journey. It was not until March 2003, after returning from my successful and enjoyable trip, that I began to need medicine for my liver again, but much less than before; and this is still the case today. Since my return I have instituted a weekly juice day in memory of the 21-day process, which suits me very well. I am once again enjoying my vegan and high-quality biodynamic food and appreciate the meals I prepare with care and gratitude.

Looking back, the process of gaining nourishment from light remains a powerful soul experience. It has given me new and most valuable vigour for life after the difficult time I had in taking leave of my teaching work after my seventieth birthday. The parting put great strain on my psychological and physical health which I have been able to overcome with medical help, with cranio-sacral massage, with the assistance of friends as well as with the healing help of the light process. So I am filled with much gratitude for the wise guidance of my destiny and for the beneficent effect of the light process which, I believe, continues to work in a helpful way.

Gertrud Müller

4

The main aim: to conduct well-founded scientific studies

by Thomas Stöckli

We have been concerned from the outset that investigations of the phenomenon of receiving nourishment from light should be carried out in accordance with strict scientific criteria. What form this might take remained open. The simplest method would be to lock up the person being investigated and keep a watch to ensure that he or she really does not eat anything. But how long can such an experiment be allowed to last? And with the scientific community being fundamentally mistrusting of such a person, how justifiable would it be to create conditions that are even more stringent than solitary confinement? For in addition to artificial light being switched on day and night and the necessary permanent guard, the person would have to be attached to an array of measuring instruments. It is not surprising, therefore, that it took many months before permission to conduct the experiment could be granted by the relevant ethical committee despite the fact that the individual undergoing the tests – Michael Werner – had freely decided that he wanted the investigations to go ahead.

But now the first important step has been taken. An initial scientific project in the form of a single-case study has been conducted by a university. Subject to strictly defined and controlled conditions an individual has lived without food of any kind for ten days under permanent medical, physiological and psychological observation and supervision. Since the scientific evaluation and interpretation of the results have not yet been made available,* we here present the subjective although very meticulous and detailed account prepared by Werner himself. This will provide critical readers with some basis upon which they may form their own opinion as to the possible evidential and scientific relevance of the experiment.

* See further on pages 215–219.

Personal report on the case study

by Michael Werner

Michael Werner's original diary entries made during the October 2004 study of 'nourishment without food'

More than two years ago a friend of mine, a physician, asked me whether I would be prepared to participate in a scientific study of my way of life. He himself would be happy to take on the scientific co-ordination and supervision as the study's director. Since I had already been thinking along the same lines I agreed immediately.

Regarding the design of the study we quickly realized that the best we could do as a first step would be to prove that my way of living was *not a matter of fasting*. We then soon agreed on an experiment lasting about ten days during which the practice of taking no food at all would be kept under strict observation. In addition every meaningful medical test and measurement that could practically be carried out would be undertaken. The purpose of the experiment would be to arrive at definite questions to which there were as yet no scientific answers or which had not yet even been asked, without making ourselves the laughing stock of the scientific community. We felt this design to be tenable and acceptable to medical and university circles including the ethics committee, and this did indeed prove to be the case.

After a great deal of preparatory effort we finally received the go-ahead from the ethics committee. Thereafter everything went very quickly, since we had long been well prepared for the work to begin. It had been up to us to find the necessary finance, and we were grateful to have this generously secured by the Asta Blumenfeldt Foundation at Dornach, Switzerland. We had also found a suitable location for the experiment: a special room in the intensive care department of a Swiss hospital providing round-the-clock CCTV surveillance and all the other necessary conditions aimed at ensuring strict abstinence from any intake of food.

So this is it! I'm on the train from Basle to the Swiss interior. It's 6 o'clock in the morning, dark and cold. I'm due at the hospital at 8.30. I have two suitcases, heavy mainly on account of many books, lap-top, a small stereo player and lots of classical music CDs. For ten days I shall be unable to leave my room, unable to open the window and, for better or for worse, stuck with the hospital's internal air-conditioning. And of course I cannot have any visitors. I wonder what all this will be like in practice. Well, I shall have to put up with it; it's what I wanted.

At the main station, somewhat flustered and anxious, I look for the bus-stop. Things are really getting close now – thank goodness!

And then I arrive at the hospital.

Day 1

A first nice surprise at the reception desk. When I ask the way to the intensive-care ward the receptionist enquires politely: 'Who do you have an appointment with?' She can't imagine anyone happily setting off for voluntary incarceration in intensive care.

The doctor in charge comes to collect me; I am warmly welcomed with a comforting lack of embarrassment and taken to the intensive-care ward on the third floor. It's new, modern and thus perhaps a little austere, but bright and comfortable. A friendly nurse conducts me to my room. And then it hits me: I shall not be leaving here for the next ten days! The room is unusually large but has only one relatively small window looking out onto a row of treetops clothed in autumn colours. The catch has been removed to prevent my opening it. So I shall indeed be dependent on the ventilation provided by the air-conditioning.

Like a space capsule, the rear wall of the room is covered with measuring instruments; not a very comforting sight. There's a small wash basin and a little wardrobe on the opposite wall. Well, of course, this is an intensive-care ward, so no shower, no bath, no toilet. Personal hygiene as in olden times. In the corner is a stand with a wide-angle camera – Big Brother says 'hello'. It'll be switched on round the clock and record my every move on tape. This means the light will have to stay on all night so that the camera can see me which probably won't trouble me much since I usually sleep like a hibernating bear. Alas, there's no writing table, and my tactful enquiry draws a blank stare – this is, after all, an intensive care ward! Never mind, I shall make do and misappropriate the dining table instead.

I unpack my suitcases. The doctor in charge minutely examines every item, like a bad day at an international border-crossing. I might have brought in some food, perhaps astronauts' provisions or something similar. But I don't mind. My cases are deposited outside the room and the planned programme commences immediately.

First comes a routine examination by the department head on duty, from top to toe, in every detail. Everything appears to be in order. Then come what are to be daily standard investigations: weight, temperature, blood pressure and oxygen saturation; and the taking of a copious amount of blood. I am well used to the latter, but I've never seen so many sample bottles waiting to be filled in one session. This is really new to me: 80–90 ml are taken this morning for every imaginable test. Fortunately this amount of blood is only to be taken on the first, sixth and tenth days, but on the others it will still be 40–50 ml every time. For cardiac and circulatory observation I am then permanently attached to the ECG machine by means of three electrodes on my upper torso. So I shall be stuck with these wires and this 'dog lead' for the next ten days. There will be no escape, for this would immediately set off the alarm in the nurses' station. Thank goodness the cable just about reaches as far as the wash basin.

From now on, at hourly(!) intervals, day and night, a member of staff will take my blood pressure and measure the oxygen saturation of my blood. Presumably this is to ensure and record the fact that my condition is regularly checked by someone. At night these checks will be done automatically, which means that the blood pressure cuff and pulse oxymeter for measuring oxygen saturation will remain attached. At least I won't be bothered by unnecessary fiddling about while I sleep, but it will involve having a further two leads attached.

Left alone for a few minutes I take some deep breaths. But almost immediately a smart young woman arrives with a large case and a trolley full of equipment. Her job is to collect calorimetric data on the first, sixth and tenth days. I have to lie down on the bed and then I disappear for 15 minutes under a tightly sealed plastic hood: my breath is being investigated. The inhaled and exhaled air is analysed and the respiratory quotient is determined; a measure for my basal metabolism as well as its quality. This, too, has been done to me before, so I'm not alarmed.

Finally comes a brief measuring of the electrical resistance of my body between the right foot and right hand to determine the composition of my body with regard to water, fat and fat-free tissue mass.

Hardly is this over when there is another knock on the door. A young, likeable doctor (with whom I shall be having many interesting conversations over the coming days) attaches me to a machine that is to measure my pulse/respiratory rate over the next 24 hours. Another three electrodes on my chest and yet another lead that like all the others is permanently on the lookout for an opportunity to get caught on something or tangle with colleagues. Luckily this one doesn't end in some distant apparatus but in a small box the size of a packet of cigarettes that now dangles from my stomach for 24 hours. In addition, however, another lead emerges from said small box. It is connected to a plug that ends up in my nostril where it measures the temperature of my breath. An additional small wire in front of my mouth constantly determines my breathing rate. Surprisingly I get used to this quite soon. This additional measurement is fortunately only to be taken for the first 24 hours.

Next I fill in four(!) psychological questionnaires which contain some very in-depth questions. I'm beginning to feel like a guinea pig in a pharmacological research establishment, except that I'm expected to fill in the forms myself.

Then at midday my first go on the ergometer, a kind of hometrainer bike that calculates and displays the amount of energy used per training unit. Since I like and am used to quite a bit of exercise it has been agreed in advance at my request that I shall be having 30 minutes of this exercise twice a day. Initially I aim for approx. 100 kJ per session, which amounts to a cycle ride of 12–13 km. Having been handicapped recently by a nasty cut on the sole of one foot which has prevented me from taking any kind of exercise, I'm not very fit at present. But this session does me good and helps make my little 'intensive cage' almost bearable.

In the afternoon the team who are to measure my autonomic nervous system arrives. They are accompanied by the deputy director of the study with whom I have so far only spoken on the telephone. For a short while a further handful of electrodes is added to the existing six. Between bouts of measuring I am subjected to an interesting psychological endurance test which is intentionally designed to put me under stress and succeeds in doing so.

From 5 to 6 p.m. I then enjoy my first, well-earned, rest. I listen to Beethoven, the first and second symphonies, and feel reconciled to the world once more. After this I talk to the director of the study on the telephone. He happens to be abroad but is easily able to coordinate and take care of everything from afar. And up to now everything has indeed gone as planned.

At 7.30 p.m. the duty cardiologist arrives to make a detailed initial investigation of everything that falls under his speciality. He thoroughly checks my heart and circulation. Everything is in good order. While he works we carry on a very intensive, open and interesting conversation about how I obtain nourishment.

After the evening 30 minutes on the ergometer I've finally had enough. I listen to Beethoven's third and fourth symphonies before going to bed. Despite all the cables and electrodes I quickly fall asleep at around midnight. Even the hourly inflation of the blood-pressure cuff makes little impression on me.

Day 2

I wake up well rested after four hours of sound sleep. My electronic trappings have hardly disturbed me at all. I get up at 5 and start the day with meditation, listening to music and reading.

The hourly blood pressure and oxygen saturation readings remain virtually constant; so everything's alright. Throughout the study these basal readings remain 'boringly' constant, staying within the normal range and showing me to be perfectly well. Apart from the brief periods on the ergometer and when I sleep my pulse is always between 80 and 60 beats per minute, my blood pressure at 130–110 over 80–60, and my oxygen saturation at 99–95 per cent (with a reading of over 92 per cent being desirable).

At 7 I mount the ergometer again and ride a distance of 12 km. Although this is strenuous and unaccustomed I notice immediately and clearly that it does me good.

The daily check-up takes place at 9: blood, this time only about 40 ml, total urine of the day before, and weight, temperature and blood pressure. The morning runs smoothly and I can concentrate a bit on my own projects.

The young physician from the university who fixed me up yesterday for the pulse/respiratory rate check comes at 11 and relieves me of the equipment. He slips the chip into his computer and explains it all to me in detail. At first sight there appears to be something unusual about my sleep pattern; we shall see whether this is repeated on Day 5. When he has finished we have a long, agreeable and far-reaching conversation about our views on the limitations of modern medicine, its prospects and possibilities.

A neurologist appears at 1 p.m. for his first check. Apart from a restriction of the reflexes in my left leg – obviously a consequence of a recent operation on a vertebra – everything is in order.

The X-ray department marches in punctually at 3 with a huge mobile machine. (For security reasons, i.e. so that I don't somehow manage to snatch any food on the way, all examinations have to take place in my room.) Now my intestines are X-rayed. This serves to discount the possibility that I might have ingested some food reserves before the beginning of the study that could now be providing me with nourishment. Of course I hadn't. Later I hear that my intestines are completely empty, that there are also no faecal residues and that there is an unusually small amount of gas.

In the early evening I have a very pleasant personal talk with the medical head of the department before I climb onto my ergometer to keep myself more or less fit.

After everything I've experienced with medics and other scientists over the last 3 years in connection with the subject of living on light, the atmosphere here in the hospital is strikingly open-minded and comfortingly uncritical. Nevertheless even here I find myself up against the usual reservations and mis-understandings fuelled by the excessive scepticism of scientists who subscribe to the motto: What I don't understand I don't believe. Added to this is the understandable though mistaken idea, which most of the people I meet here have, that my reason for coming here is to demonstrate that I am capable of going without food for 10 days. When I say that I have not eaten anything for the last three-and-a-half years and that this is 'normal' for me, my statement is either ignored or not acknowledged.

What has been noticeable today is that I haven't been thirsty at all in spite of having a very dry mouth – no doubt because of the air-conditioning. There is a danger that I might lose some weight. Perhaps this is why I've been feeling somewhat limp all day. After a quiet evening I go to bed at 11 p.m. and immediately fall deeply asleep.

Day 3

It's 2 o'clock in the morning. After sleeping for 3 hours I wake up having slept long enough. I listen to music and read. I still don't feel thirsty. Having had slightly sour eructations since yesterday I've decided to change from the herb tea provided to some camomile and fennel tea. I feel a slight pressure in my ears like coming down from the mountains by car or landing after a flight.

In addition to my mouth being dry my voice is also slightly hoarse. This might be caused by tissue dehydration and wouldn't be a good sign. So I decide to force myself to drink larger amounts of tea and mineral water.

At the 9 a.m. check-up it turns out that I have indeed lost a considerable amount of weight: 800 grammes. This is rather a lot, so I must drink more!

Then I get on the ergometer for my morning ride. Still feeling rather feeble I soon notice that my performance is well below par. I'm determined to reach the set 100 kJ in 30 minutes so for the last few metres I force myself to do better. As a result my pulse rockets to 159 beats a minute which in turn sets off the alarm and causes hectic activity to break out in my room; but I succeed. After that I'm completely done in and allow myself the relaxing luxury of a Vivaldi CD.

I'm doing better at drinking today, especially after diluting the tea a lot with sparkling mineral water.

In the evening I talk to the study director on the telephone as usual, but apart from the surprising loss of weight there's nothing special to report.

I feel tired quite early, so go to bed at 10 p.m. and immediately fall asleep.

Day 4
I wake up at half an hour past midnight, having slept deeply for only two-and-a-half hours. I listen to music for a while, and read a bit. Then I decide to lie down again to avoid bringing on the backache, and doze till about 5. Because of all the cables I unfortunately can't do my morning back exercises which I have come to appreciate very much.

I find that this is the second day of my saliva being unpleasantly viscous. I try not swallowing it but spitting it into a soft cloth which I rinse out from time to time. Soon I discover that this was a good idea. The experiment with the sparkling water, which otherwise I don't like very much and which usually doesn't really agree with me, has also had excellent results. I can now drink appropriate amounts without feeling too much aversion. In fact all in all I feel a great deal better today than I have been feeling for the past three days. Although it's still a bit hoarse, my voice has also improved noticeably.

During the daily check-up at 9 a.m. I'm found to have lost a bit more weight since yesterday, but the amount is so small that I'm confident of my condition becoming stabilized.

I have plenty of peace and quiet today, as there's nothing on the programme except another four psychological test questionnaires to be filled in. The study director comes to see me in the afternoon. I've known him well for many years and we spend a few pleasant hours talking about interesting things.

The evening is quiet, almost boring, and I go to bed at 10.30 feeling surprisingly tired.

Day 5

By 2 a.m. I've had enough sleep. Having greeted the early morning with Mozart's Clarinet Concerto I go back to bed and doze till 5 in order to rest my back, which is still sometimes quite painful. I'm certainly rather restricted in my movements here, and I do want to prevent the onset of some serious backache.

I'm still making sure to drink plenty of liquid, and this is no longer a problem at all. I feel markedly 'heavier', the pressure in my ears has gone, my voice is now almost normal, and my saliva is once again comfortably fluid.

The 9 o'clock check-up brings a good and important confirmation: I've gained some weight. This is excellent, since a continued loss of weight might fatally call the whole experiment

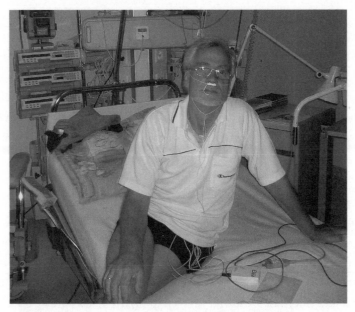

Keeping a constant check on heart function (ECG) and respiratory rate.

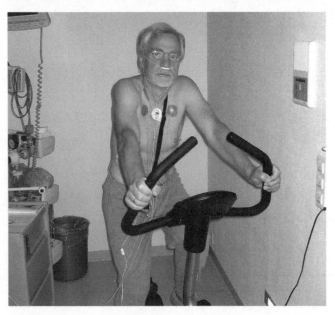

Daily exercise on the ergometer to measure additional use of calories.

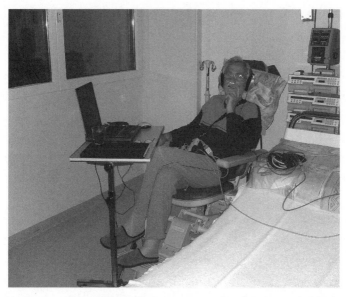

Taking time off to relax and listen to music. 'You have to make the best of things.'

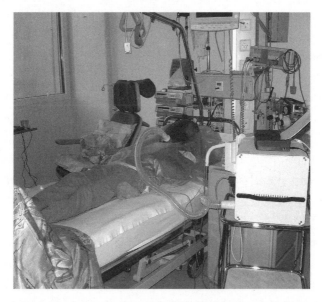

Measuring the composition of exhaled air to determine basic calorimetric data.

into question, in keeping with the motto: 'He doesn't eat, so as you can see, he's digesting his own body — just as happens in every case of fasting.'

Time for my daily personal hygiene session. After sponging myself down from head to toe while avoiding the cables with some difficulty, I now have a nurse rather perilously washing my hair. For a shower and bath fanatic like me this feels truly marvellous. In this connection I should point out, though, that since ceasing to eat I have been less sweaty and my general 'pong' has been a great deal more civilized.

A comfortable afternoon. It's raining and windy outside and people tell me the weather is a lot colder. I read, listen to music, work at my computer, talk on the telephone and watch a bit of tennis on the television. The study director visits me again in the late afternoon. We discuss the results so far. Since my weight now appears to be stable, the biggest problem has been defused for the time being. But some of the laboratory readings are still unusually high. The next few days will show where this is leading.

On account of the laboratory results and the uncertainty about my weight I've reduced my aim for the ergometer from 100 to 60 kJ per 30 minutes. This makes life a good deal more pleasant and less strenuous, and I shall continue like this for a few days.

After a short but very nice conversation with the department head I'm free for the rest of the evening. I'm tired at around 11 p.m. and go to bed.

I meet a good many people, also here in the hospital, who, while not exactly rejecting the idea of living on light, nevertheless remain rather unimpressed by the phenomenon. For a proper awareness of this process and its true significance to become established perhaps it will be necessary for a kind of 'critical mass' to be reached. There is obviously still a long way to go before this happens. I don't mean a 'critical mass' with regard to the number of individuals practising it, but a 'critical mass' with regard to the amount of information that is available.

Surprisingly tonight I'm having difficulty falling asleep, which is very rare for me. After several attempts and getting quite agitated, which makes me cross and shows how spoilt I am in this respect, I finally drop off at around half past midnight.

Day 6

I wake up at 4 a.m. having had enough sleep. After my customary rather hampered morning ablutions I begin the day with Beethoven.

This is going to be a busy day as all the measurements carried out in this study now fall due at once. After my session on the ergometer everything happens in quick succession. First comes a brief but very intense and open conversation with the deputy director of the study. With his well-trained physician's eye he looks me over challengingly as if to say: 'Well, after 6 days of not eating surely there must be something noticeable to observe.'

Then a smart young lady arrives to do the calorimetry. Once again I disappear for 15 minutes under the blue plastic hood well-sealed with the help of plastic aprons so that the composition of my breath can be analysed. Then come the four electrodes for the impedance measurement of the comparative amounts of water, fat and fat-free tissue mass in my body.

In between all this the daily extraction of 40 ml of blood and the daily temperature and weight checks have taken place. My weight has been practically constant now for the last 4 days.

Then my autonomic nervous system is investigated by means of numerous electrodes attached to my upper torso. Two young scientific assistants from the university are taking care of me and my nerves, or at least the autonomous ones. The technology, namely the computer, is playing up today, so it takes about half an hour to get a proper reading. Meanwhile another three electrodes are added for determining the pulse/respiratory rate. Again the technology plays up, but in the end everything gets done.

After this I meet the deputy department head who will now be on duty during the day. We quickly get into a very interesting conversation about the phenomenon of living on light. With two or three direct questions he hits the nail on the head without displaying any kind of embarrassment. An exceedingly satisfying, though rather rare, experience.

Then comes a well-earned pause in the proceedings interrupted only by the hourly blood-pressure and oxygen saturation checks. At 2.30 p.m. the X-ray department arrives again with its alarming apparatus. This time my intestines are X-rayed while I lie on my side and on my back to make sure I haven't ingested any food by some miraculous means.

The rest of the day is taken up with the routine examinations, and some work, reading, listening to music and talking on the telephone.

I go to bed at 11 p.m., glad of the opportunity to stretch my limbs at last.

Day 7
Again I only sleep for two hours, and even these are interrupted by a sudden urgent need to urinate. But I'm wide awake and have evidently had enough sleep.

However, I remain in bed till 5, close my eyes and listen to music. I'm accustomed to these very short bouts of sleep and know that my eyes often start to smart and my back aches if I spend too little time lying down.

After the morning routine (60 ml of blood are taken today) I have another conversation with the deputy study director. My weight is the same as the past few days and so has been practically constant for 5 days. Regarding my initial weight loss he tells me that, probably in connection with this, the level of keto bodies in my urine is up. This points to fat combustion(!). Yesterday the calorimetry showed a fat quota of about 16 per cent (in men readings between 10 and 30 per cent are normal). If this reading is confirmed on Day 10, this may be a reason for extending the experiment by a few days. Although this might necessitate shifting a few appointments I immediately agree in principle since the questions now raised might provide a way of throwing light on the 'mechanism' of living on light.

In the late morning, after 24 hours of continuous measurements, I am once again relieved of the electrodes that serve to determine my pulse/respiratory rate. The young doctor who, apart from all his usual duties, also kindly supplies me with a copy of the daily newspaper each morning, once more explains the method and purpose of the readings of the past 24 hours. They clearly show the transitions between the sleeping, resting and active phases. Once again there are some curious anomalies during my 2-hour sleep. I wonder what the final evaluations will show.

A quiet afternoon during which I enjoy Mozart's Requiem followed by the merriment of Vivaldi's Concerti Grossi. It hasn't stopped raining and looks so miserably wet out of doors that even inside my climatized isolation capsule I feel the need to put on something warmer. It's rather fortunate not to be allowed out; instead I can work here in peace and quiet.

A long talk on the telephone with the study director in the early evening. Having thought the matter over, I'm not too keen on extending the study but would tend to argue instead for a follow-up involving detailed observation and measurement of any interesting and striking parameters a little while after the planned conclusion of the study on Day 10. Of course it wouldn't be as easy as it is here in the hospital to ensure that I don't eat anything. But frequent blood checks coupled perhaps with X-rays of the intestines etc. could be accepted as a more or less reliable guarantee of my abstinence from food. We shall have to see.

I am happy and grateful for the satisfactory way in which the experiment is proceeding both as to the external circumstances and the good state I find myself in − the latter despite the extreme restriction of movement, the permanent CCTV surveillance, the complete lack of fresh air and the constant artificial light including during the night. The satisfactory situation as a whole is surely also due to the attitude of the personnel who are without exception friendly and positive, but also to the many people who are thinking of me, and the helping and healing forces of light which are making their beneficial contribution in these unusual circumstances.

I retire at 11 p.m. and as usual fall asleep quickly.

Day 8

I sleep for two-and-a-half hours with one short interruption, but as before I don't get up until 5 when I begin my usual morning routine.

After the ergometer session and before the thorough morning check-up at 9 a.m. I have another talk with the deputy study director. They want to do an extra daily check on my weight to get a clearer picture of what is going on. I rather doubt that this will mean much at this late stage. They are also tending quite strongly towards adding a further 3 days to the study in order to

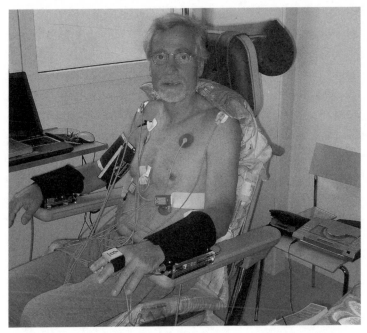

Wired up to the limit: measuring functions of the autonomic nervous system.

collect further readings regarding my body-weight and more information from the calorimetry.

This morning my weight is slightly down on yesterday; so I share their curiosity as to what the second reading of the day will be.

Otherwise this is 'not my day'. I don't fancy the idea of staying on for a further 3 days since this will unavoidably cause considerable stress in my work during the following week.

I do some reading in between getting on the phone a few times to sort out my appointments log-jam as best I can. Unfortunately I don't have access to the internet or e-mail here. At 6.30 p.m. the second weigh-in takes place. I've lost another 0.5 kg. I'm not too surprised as I have been passing unusual amounts of urine since this morning and have once again had very little desire to drink. According to my notes this alone would account for a weight difference of 0.6 kg. Admittedly, though, this further loss of weight makes everything more difficult or, for sceptics, simpler.

Because of the unusual nature of my cardiac variables during my short phases of sleep at night I am to be attached once more this evening to the machine for measuring my pulse/respiratory rate. This will give us a further night's readings in case it becomes necessary to reproduce the phenomenon. The young doctor handling this has to come back late in the evening because of this. We have a long and very good talk about the possibilities and significance of living on light. From my point of view a comforting end to the day.

I go to bed at 11.30 p.m. and sleep deeply for an hour.

Day 9

I wake up at half past midnight, listen to music and doze for a while. Towards morning I sleep for about another hour and begin my day at 5 a.m. with a rather laborious shave.

The morning check-up reveals that my weight is the same as yesterday evening – so the mystery continues.

Later in the morning I join the doctor in charge in examining the night-time readings of the pulse/respiratory rate. The strange symptom of the unusually narrow range of pulse frequency during sleep has occurred again. Since today is anyway the day when I am to be wired up for a 24-hour period, this will give us a further opportunity to check this anomaly. During these 24-hour readings I have been instructed to fit in five 15-minute sessions of absolute bodily and as far as I am able also mental rest at specified times during the day. A comprehensive study comprising a large number of healthy test subjects is ongoing at present with the intention of discovering whether this method of obtaining readings and its results can supply basic information on the state of health of the persons being examined.

The afternoon follows the usual pattern. I'm starting to feel bored. And I'm beginning to be apprehensive about perhaps really having to stay in my 'monastic cell' for an extra three days.

The evening weigh-in is disappointing since I have again lost some weight. Perhaps I'm still drinking too little given the very dry air in this room. Well, it's too late now. I shall try to investigate this in peace when I get home by simulating the conditions here as well as I can. The disappointing matter of this fluctuation of my weight will probably mean that the whole study has become irrelevant as to its original purpose, so we should work towards bringing it to a close tomorrow. On the other hand I don't want to be the 'spoilsport' since this might have an unfavourable influence on the subsequent interpretation.

During our evening talk shortly before he goes home, the department head tells me that my standard blood and urine readings are all in order except for the elevated level of keto bodies in the urine.

After making a few phone calls and reinstating the machine for measuring my pulse/respiratory rate (which I had accidentally switched off during the resting phase) I go to bed at 11 p.m.

Day 10
After two periods of sleep totalling three-and-a-half hours I get up at 5 a.m. and begin my morning routine, perhaps for the last time in this setting. I've gone over everything many times in my mind and am still inclined to think it would be better to finish the experiment today as planned. The data we have gathered — which includes much that is positive and interesting — would

not look fundamentally different after a further three days. And the same goes for whatever we have not so far achieved.

Today all the checks set up as intermittent measurements for the comprehensive research programme of the study will be repeated once more. In other words, this is likely to be another rather stressful morning.

The daily checks begin at 9 a.m. My weight hasn't changed since yesterday – which is rather a relief. As on the first day, the blood taken will once again amount to a rather alarming 80–90 ml. Account will surely have to be taken of this in the balances of all the other vital blood constituents, for added to the regular blood samples taken it amounts to a good half litre, which alone adds up to 0.5 kg in weight loss. And this takes no account of other vital constituents lost for which the body itself has to compensate immediately.

9.30 a.m. The nice young lady of Day 1, in another all-black outfit, arrives with the calorimetry equipment. After a short pause for setting up the apparatus and the stipulated 15-minute rest period I once again disappear under the plastic hood which is thoroughly sealed all round. My basal energy conversion is determined via the respiratory rate and subsequently also the composition of my body mass. This enables relatively accurate deductions to be made regarding the type of metabolism, e.g. whether combustion is more via carbohydrates, fat or protein (muscle) mass. I gather from the brief subsequent discussion of the readings that today, Day 10, there is a slightly lower reading for my basal metabolism and a little less fat metabolism as compared with Day 6. After this comes the impedance reading by means of which the comparative water, fat, fat-free and muscle masses can be established. Since calculation of the data requires a special computer programme, there is no immediate information regarding today's readings. A direct comparison between Day 1 and Day 6 showed that the fat content had decreased by about 1.5%, the fat-free tissue mass had remained practically constant, and the muscle portion had increased slightly. The latter is unusual and cannot be explained; perhaps an error in the reading.

Next come the tests on the autonomic nervous system. Via 8 or 9 additional electrodes the electrical impulses on and/or in the upper abdomen are recorded. Ten-minute readings are taken twice, once after a 15-minute rest period and then in the recovery period immediately following a psychological stress test. The results or trends of these tests are not yet available. Since the method and significance of these readings is new and unclear to me, I am all the more agog as to the final evaluation.

During a very interesting talk with the department head which followed, the expected call from the study director comes through. The question is whether to continue for a further three days or bring the study to an end today as planned. After a short weighing-up of the pros and cons we decide to finish today. An additional three days would probably not have answered or refined the questions arising but only made them more obvious. Finally I fill in the familiar four psychological questionnaires. Then I pack my things and take leave of the ward staff.

Leaving the hospital I revel in the fresh air like an astronaut returning to earth. The weather is wonderful as I dawdle to the rail station. The bustle on the streets seems strange but I enjoy it. I'm returning from a strenuous trip that has also been impressive and interesting.

During the whole of the study I found that the relevant spiritual powers were quite reserved in offering me assistance and suggestions regarding living on light. This gives me a good, indeed an almost confident feeling that I am on the right path, a path of personal choice and responsibility for myself, that is in keeping with our time.

Whether living on light works or does not work and whether it is appropriate for a particular person depends mainly on the positive will that one is able or prepared to muster. This involves active, courageous and confident open-mindedness and a willingness to approach the unknown and the unbelievable. The rest is down to practice in faith, hope and love for life.

Preliminary conclusions

by Michael Werner

One important general aim of this study was to try and open up at least a small chink in the solid armour of today's academic medical world. Whether this has succeeded or will succeed remains to be seen when the comprehensive final evaluation of all the data is published.*

That a human being can live without eating, can feel well and function normally under normal circumstances may seem plausible to medical doctors who are open-minded, observant and innovative, just as it is to other ordinary people who are willing to accept the facts. But official medical science with its established and of course also well-tried methods still has no truck with claims as seemingly audacious as: 'The human being can live without eating!' I am all the more grateful to all those who have helped make this study possible in the first place. It has been necessary to overcome many small and large obstacles and to replace prejudice with trust.

It is not for me to undertake a scientific evaluation of the study and I do not intend to attempt such a thing here. On the one hand I lack the scientific competence and probably also the necessary neutrality. And on the other hand the data has not yet been adequately evaluated and interpreted, so that there would be too much speculation. In addition it is obvious that until the evaluation is published in a recognized medical journal I am not

---

* See Afterword.

permitted to pass on any specific information relevant to that evaluation. So the following remarks will not go beyond generalities and some entirely personal comments in order not to anticipate the fundamental discussion on the study results. Looking back at my experiences during those 10 days I realize that in any future investigations of this nature some fundamental aspects will have to be improved or reconsidered.

Two factors had a strong bearing on the experiment and are therefore especially worth mentioning. The first concerns a seeming detail of the general setting. In order to ensure that I could not obtain any food from outside, the windows were completely sealed, shutting out any natural fresh air, which meant that the air I breathed came exclusively from the air-conditioning system and was thus partially recycled and had no doubt had any organisms filtered out. It was devoid of the water droplets present in natural air, an impairment which I found very uncomfortable and also debilitating. With a little extra ingenuity and care this could easily be improved on, so every effort should be made to do this in any future studies.

The second factor concerns myself or any other future candidate. I underestimated the effect of abandoning my accustomed lifestyle on entering the necessarily cramped circumstances of the study with all the restrictions they imposed. So any future subject would be well advised to make much more careful preparations for the experiment.

I nevertheless hope that the study will provide a point of departure for further investigations and will move one person or another among the scientific fraternity to follow up new and unusual ideas.

A critical appraisal

by Thomas Stöckli

Michael Werner's description clearly shows up a systemic contradiction inherent in the study: in order to prove that an individual can survive on nourishment derived from vital energy, present-day science requires the individual in question to be rigorously isolated from almost all such energy. The conclusion then reached is that instead of receiving nourishment as claimed the individual was merely fasting. This is a logical conclusion that should not be found surprising, for it was indeed akin to fasting if he was shut up in a sterile, artificially lit and ventilated room which isolated him from all natural carriers of life (water droplets in the air, human company and natural exercise). Prior to the study this was insufficiently clear to all those involved including above all Michael Werner himself.

The study is thus open to various interpretations. On the one hand it could be said to show that it is impossible for a human being to be fed by 'light' and that this is always merely a form of fasting. Or, on the other hand, it can show that in an artificial and sterile environment inimical to life it is impossible to be fed directly by vital energy, i.e. light. Both these interpretations are possible, so the reader is free to decide which of the two he or she favours.

For the sake of overcoming today's one-sided materialism there will always be calls for open-mindedness towards a more comprehensive, holistic and spiritual understanding of the world. It would be a contradiction in terms to accept a spiritual view of the world served up to us on a plate full of external proofs. Spirituality today is neither spiritualism nor materialized miracles; it always draws on one's own critical faculties and active thinking. If we did not bring these into play we could easily fall for any kind of magic, whether it be that of accepting scientific results we do not understand or that of naively believing in outdated miracles.

Michael Werner is one of those who strive for a new and wider understanding of science while remaining fully aware that his own knowledge, experiences and observations are also limited. He describes a phenomenon without immediately feeling the need to prove it by means of ready-made theories. Instead he maintains an inquiring, open-minded research attitude that is free of any preconceived doctrinal opinions, a frame of mind that is surely appropriate in the face of phenomena such as that of living on light.

PART TWO: REFLECTIONS

5

In place of dogma: science that is critical and relevant

by Thomas Stöckli

It has to be stated that Michael Werner does not in any way seek to make propaganda for the possibility of receiving nourishment from light. Whenever he lectures he states quite categorically: 'My concern is not a question of ceasing to eat but of beginning to think in a different way.'

This is also the motivation that lies behind the publication of this book. We are first and foremost concerned to give a serious description of a phenomenon for which an explanation has not yet been found and which therefore bothers and provokes us. It is not a matter of creating a sensation but of giving a straightforward account of facts that are unusual and should therefore be called into question.

Scientific scepticism is a part of this but it is important not to apply the prejudices of popular science to new phenomena. Unfortunately ill-considered dogmatic beliefs do to a large extent dominate even mainstream science, and it is from this that generally recognized ideas about the world originate. Interestingly, however, the most up-to-date discoveries of physics, the science that researches the material world, are themselves now calling into question those very same outdated ideas. Thus Hanns-Peter Dürr, professor of physics, has come to the conclusion: 'We can no longer comprehend even matter itself. It is not that we cannot understand the soul with the help of our concept of matter;

startlingly, matter itself has suddenly begun to behave "just like" the soul.'*

All of a sudden the thing we are most sure about is snatched from us, namely matter as the basis of today's 'materialism', and as if this were not enough it is also linked directly to soul and spirit. However, this insight has not yet taken hold in our everyday consciousness because we still continue to experience the everyday world as consisting of solid matter that feels firm, and because we interpret our sensory impressions by means of specific thought constructs – more from habit, however, than by thinking independently. Scientists, meanwhile, are beginning to question the old doctrine concerning the 'eternal laws of nature':

> The presumption today is that we are living in an open, evolu-
> tionary universe. So it is high time to begin questioning laws that
> are supposed to remain constant for ever. In my opinion it makes
> more sense to imagine the laws of nature as rules which change
> and develop hand in hand with the universe ... When certain
> patterns are constantly repeated, habits become impressed into
> nature's memory in a way that makes them seem like eternal
> laws. But interesting things happen in connection with new
> phenomena, for example when a new chemical substance is
> crystallized, when a dog or a rat learns a new behaviour, when
> humans adopt new ideas and new ways of doing things.
> According to my theory, such phenomena will occur more
> frequently and more easily all over the world the more often they
> have been repeated.†

This is how Rupert Sheldrake put it in an interview. With a PhD in biology he has for years been researching phenomena that have been dismissed as 'inexplicable' by conventional science.

---

* Dürr, 2001.
† Quoted in von Lüpke, 2003.

What does the chemist Dr Werner say about nourishment from food or from light?

Food provides the body with the life forces it requires. Might it not in fact be possible for the body to receive those life forces in a new way through light as an alternative to the usual method of eating solid food? For clearly, nourishment is not solely a matter of absorbing physical substances, since imponderables such as information and the energy of light and heat, as well as psychological and spiritual influences, also have a direct part to play. And it is equally clear that we do not actually know how the transformation of the substances we eat comes about. As a chemist, Michael Werner has this to say:

We humans are constantly balancing the substances in our body in a flow equilibrium, i.e. with our food we normally absorb solid substances such as minerals, carbohydrates, fats and proteins as well as large amounts of water. A portion of all this is immediately excreted again via the intestines and bladder. The smaller remaining portion is processed by means of very comprehensive and complicated biochemical metabolic chains in the lymph, blood and liver etc. at organic, cellular and molecular levels. In addition there is respiration which involves taking in oxygen and expelling carbon dioxide and water. These processes enable our body constantly to change and transform itself. Hair, nails, flakes of skin, sweat, but also symptoms of growth and ageing, bear obvious witness to this.

All this is described in its essentials by the ideas of modern physiology. And it is further enlarged on by what the spiritual scientist Rudolf Steiner had to say regarding the processes of assimilation and metamorphosis.

There are greater and lesser, faster and slower cycles that maintain us in our physical life through their constant flow. When light provides our nourishment these processes are re-formed, being changed for the most part at the starting point of the flow equilibrium, for they are evidently essential for life. Living on light therefore signifies not only the opening up of a new source of energy – something that is not too difficult to imagine – but also the condensation of substances. Without this supposition it is not possible to explain the measurable balances of substances. The mere fact that one can maintain a stable body weight for months while taking no food at all and only minimal amounts of liquid cannot be explained on the basis of traditional ideas. Yet it is perfectly possible to live in this way without any problems. And, astonishingly, the very extensive physiological data accumulated thus far do not suggest any irregularities or unusual phenomena.

All this raises more questions than it answers. I have therefore embarked on a personal quest to get to the bottom of these questions and with this in mind to make myself available for observations and tests.

Independent thinking and research, not a personality cult

There is also a second matter in which we do not want to be misunderstood. While we hope for critical readers who think independently, and who neither cling to pre-formed scientific opinions nor open themselves naively to every New Age way of thinking, we also want to guard against any kind of personality cult. Not only does Michael Werner describe himself as an entirely average human being; that is indeed exactly what he is. In calling himself 'Mr Ordinary' he does, however, misrepresent one aspect, namely that he is one of a small minority who can live without eating solid food. As a scientist he is more surprised about this than anyone else, and he has as yet found no simple explanation, which is the very reason why he is attracted to science: it enables new realms to be researched and new theories to be developed.

So our concern here is to accept quite objectively the phenomenon of this scientist and his experiences while also seeing in them a challenge to our thinking, to our view of science, and to our current view of the world without making the mistake either of believing him naively or of rejecting the phenomenon without testing it.

In the following we give some relatively extensive quotations from the works of Rudolf Steiner as an encouragement to question everyday procedures, such as eating, and to begin thinking in entirely new ways. Among many other subjects, this advanced thinker and researcher examined these matters in detail.

Food for thought in the works of Rudolf Steiner

Early in the twentieth century during the course of his researches in spiritual science, Rudolf Steiner formulated a number of basic tenets regarding these matters which still today can help us work towards finding answers to them. Speaking in Hamburg on 27 May 1910 he said:

> There is a fundamental essence of our material earth existence out of which all matter only comes into being by a condensing process, and to the question: What is the fundamental substance of our earth existence?, spiritual science gives the answer: 'Every substance upon the earth is condensed light!' There is nothing in material existence in any form whatever which is anything but condensed light ... Wherever you reach out and touch a substance, there you have condensed, compressed light. All matter is, in its essence, light.*

---

* R. Steiner, 1995.

If the source of all matter is light, then this must also apply to the human physical body, so Steiner continued quite logically: *'Inasmuch as man is a material being, he is composed of light.'*

Based on this statement we can now try to look more closely at the matter of ingesting nourishment. In a lecture he gave on 18 July 1923 Steiner began by describing fear as an example of how psychological states affect the body and how what is physical and sense-perceptible relates to the spiritual. At the end of this lecture there is a fundamental description of the process of being nourished which is interesting and important in connection with the matter of living on light. First of all he introduced the subject by mentioning the well-known fact that over a period of about seven years the physical substance of the human body is completely renewed. In other words, all the substances are exchanged and replaced during the course of seven years. Along with nails, hair and sweat all bodily substances are continuously shed and replaced by new, 'fresh' ones.

In simple, clear and forceful lines Steiner proceeded to paint a picture of his observations and experiences concerning the way the human being takes in nourishment:

He [the human being] is all the time giving off matter and is all the time taking in new matter. People therefore think that matter comes in through the mouth and goes out again through the anus and in the urine, and the human being is a kind of tube. He takes in matter with his food, keeps it for a time and then discards it again. That is more or less how people think man is made. But the truth is that nothing of the earthly matter enters into the real human being, none at all. That is just an illusion. It is like this. If we eat potatoes, say, this is not in order to take in something from the potato. The potato is merely something which stimulates us, stimulates us in the jaw, the gullet and so on. It is active just there. And then the power develops in us to discard the potato again and, as we drive it out, the principle which builds up our body in the course of seven years approaches us from the ether, not from the solid matter. We actually do not at all build our bodies with earthly matter. We only eat the things we eat to get a stimulus ... However, the situation is that irregularities may of course occur. For if we take too much food the food stays inside us for too long. We then collect unjustifiable food in us, grow corpulent, fat, and so on. If we take in too little we do not get enough stimulus and do not take enough of what we need from the world of the spirit, from the etheric world. This is something most important ... this fact that we do not build ourselves up out of the earth and its matter but that we build ourselves up out of something that is beyond the earth. If it is the case that the whole body is renewed in seven years, the heart will also be renewed. So you no longer have the heart inside you now that you had eight years ago. It has been renewed, renewed not from the material substance of the earth but renewed out of the element that surrounds the earth in the light. Your heart is compressed light! You really and truly have a heart that is condensed sunlight. And the food you have eaten has only given the stimulus for you to compress the sunlight so far. You build up all your organs from the light-filled surroundings, and the fact that we eat, that we take in food, only means that a stimulus is given.*

With the first core statement that all matter, all substances, molecules and so on stem ultimately from light through processes of condensation or compression, and with the second description of the human being condensing the substance of his body directly out of the etheric realm of light, we are given a plausible bridge to the phenomenon of receiving nourishment

---

* R. Steiner, 2000.

from light. We are shown in principle how we might imagine the process.

However, in the course of lectures he gave on agriculture at Koberwitz in the following year, Steiner partially revised what he had said previously. In the lecture of 16 June 1924 he described the substances in the body as consisting partly of earthly matter – namely the system of nerves and senses – and partly of cosmic material – namely the system of the limbs and the metabolism. In the final analysis, therefore, the relationship between external substances and the constitution, formation and renewal of the physical body through food and the process of nourishment turns out to be somewhat more complicated and differentiated:

> The important thing is not the ... process whereby foodstuffs are taken up from outside and then deposited in the body, as people always imagine, even if they also imagine all kinds of transformations along the way ... The substances of our system of metabolism and limbs – everything constituting our intestines, limbs, muscles, bones, and so forth – do not come from the earth, but from what is absorbed out of the air and warmth above the earth. That is cosmic substantiality ... The cosmic matter is absorbed through the senses and through breathing.*

And on 20 June 1924 Steiner then described the process further in more graphic terms:

> People think nourishment consists in our eating the substances that are around us. First these go into the mouth, and then into the stomach. Then some of them are deposited in the body and some of them are excreted. Next the deposited portion is used up and also gets excreted, after which it is again replaced. People conceive of nutrition in the most superficial fashion. But the fact

---

* R. Steiner, 1993.

is that the foodstuffs taken in through the stomach do not build up our bones, muscles, and other tissues – they only build up our head. Everything that enters the body by way of the digestive organs, and is then metabolized and distributed, only provides materials to be deposited in the head, in what belongs to the nerve-sense system. On the other hand, the substances we need for building up our limbs or our metabolic organs ... do not come from the food taken in by way of our mouth and stomach; instead they are absorbed from our whole environment by means of our breathing, and even via our sensory organs. Within each human being, the following process is continually taking place: What is taken in through our stomach streams upward and is put to use in our head, while what comes from the air and the rest of our surroundings is taken in through our head – our nerve-sense system – and then streams downward to build up the organs of our digestive system or our limbs.*

Living on light – a 'message'

Since the subject of being nourished by light first became known through the book *Living on Light*, it appears that thousands of people all over the world are following this way of life. Is it true that an entirely new possibility of drawing nourishment directly from life energy has become a reality for 'perfectly ordinary people' and not only for yogis or 'saints'? We maintain that perhaps it is indeed a relatively new human capacity to be able to survive entirely on light or on life energy. Michael Werner always states quite clearly in his lectures: '*I would not speak publicly about this if I thought that I was a special case in having this capability.*'

The spiritual world does not stand still, and this potential can

---

* Ibid.

be brought to the attention of the whole of humanity by means of a single individual who adapts to this way of receiving nourishment. It is a clear and quite distinct 'message' that the human being does not live by bread alone but can indeed exist entirely without any physical food. This implies that our fixed models concerning the process of receiving nourishment are limited and thus out of date. They continue to serve as models for the majority of habits involving food but now have the tendency to tie us to an image of the human being that is entirely materialistic.

Admittedly, individuals such as Nicholas von der Flüe or Therese of Konnersreuth were proved to have 'nourished themselves by other means'. But in their time they represented a rare and special kind of human being. Now, however, it seems that a wave of new forces is beginning to manifest and pervade the physical world, so that a few decades from today it will no longer be possible to regard such phenomena as 'miracles' or indeed 'crazy ideas'. In the years to come it will be necessary for a new image of the human being and of the world to come to the fore through which this new reality will be able to create new scientific and social perspectives. As we said earlier on, our primary objective is not to make propaganda for this method of receiving nourishment but to open the way for new forces in all spheres of life so that radically new possibilities can come about for shaping life and being active in it. This is already being brought about by the breathtaking speed of technological development that is creating numerous advances which our ancestors would have regarded as 'miracles'. We are so fascinated by them that we are inclined to forget that miracles can and do also happen in everyday life and that we impose limitations on ourselves through adhering only to our customary view of the world.

> *'Rather than a universe of static certainty, the world and everything within it forms, on the material level, an uncertain and unpredictable state of pure potential and unlimited possibilities.'* (McTaggart)

Do the earth and the environment, indeed do we ourselves and our contemporaries all over the planet not need entirely new forces in order to secure life on earth and make it worth living?

And what about proofs?

Today's leading scientists already realize that we shall have to redefine entirely what we mean by understanding, perceiving and knowing: *'Exact science presupposes that it will ultimately always be possible, even in every new field of experience, to comprehend nature; but that from the start there is no consensus on what the word "comprehend" means ...'*

This statement was made by Professor Werner Heisenberg in a lecture he gave in 1953 on 'The Image of Nature in Modern Physics'. It applies equally to the matter of furnishing proof. Leading scientists have long since passed beyond the necessity for absolute proof through so-called objective experimentation. An individual initiating and carrying out an experiment influences the experiment as such and also its interpretation through the point of view from which he approaches it using the models (provisional, of course!) which he designs. Whether he trusts the data displayed on a monitor or his own direct observations, the evidence as experienced must always be combined with reason and critical, logical thinking. Evidential experience, direct perception of what is there, is the most immediate and powerful. If I see a hot stove, touch it and burn my hand, and if someone then comes along and maintains that the stove does not exist and that I cannot prove that it does, then I shall say to the doubter that my certain knowledge comes from my direct perception and that for me this counts as proof of the stove's existence.

The same can be applied to the phenomenon of being nourished by light. Because the scientist Michael Werner wanted one hundred per cent proof, he tried it himself. Anyone who wants to know but doesn't like the idea of trying it out himself can go in search of reports on the matter, or may perhaps become acquainted with someone who has done it. This, too, provides a strong form of proof, and meeting such a person can leave a lasting impression.

Michael Werner as an 'object of research'

The science of today finds Michael Werner entirely provoking, so he as a person and the circumstances of his life are likely to be scrutinized in the utmost detail.

Let us therefore begin by taking a critical look at his work environment: What do his colleagues think of him? They confirm that he is a reliable and sound manager of the institute. He is an entirely normal and appreciated colleague in his responsible position. In addition he is a scientist, a doctor of chemistry, who knows a great deal about substances and physiological processes.

And what about his health and general physical condition? As we noted earlier, Michael Werner is physically fit, does sport, goes sailing and plays tennis. With his tanned complexion and swinging gait this 56-year-old certainly does not give the impression of being a 'hunger artist'. He also has exceptional stamina, for example when travelling. He can drive from Basle to a meeting in Berlin (about 530 miles), have discussions with other participants until late into the night and then drive home again to be at work early for important business meetings.

His wife, a teacher at a Waldorf school and a warm-hearted and intelligent woman, followed the process her husband underwent with great attention in order to assess how he felt once he had changed his way of receiving nourishment. But everything has settled down and nothing much has changed as regards their family and private life, as any guest may observe. She has, however, been surprised that those among their immediate friends who know about it either cannot or do not want to deal with the subject.

Personal friends as well as academics turn a blind eye

The matter is ignored not only in private but also in the academic world where spiritual experiences are anyway viewed with scepticism. Werner has always known that he would be a living provocation as far as science was concerned but he finds this quite acceptable since the materialistic view of the world cannot be countered by theory alone. *'Although the materialistic view of the world can be countered with ideas and in theory, this is no longer sufficient in this day and age. Practical and entirely concrete proof is required. So all of a sudden even people I know quite well find me a problem.'*

Even scientists familiar with spiritual ideas are not necessarily open to the subject; indeed, one has to concede that every individual reacts in a different way. Michael Werner is experiencing the whole gamut of reactions, from interest and openness to complete rejection. 'Somehow I have the feeling that it is simply "too way out" for people. They usually ignore it. Every scientist profoundly fears having to revise his whole view of the world to which he has become so attached.'

Of course some scientists are very open, among them the physician and psychiatrist Jakob Bösch. As described in the foreword to this book, he has himself undergone an important experience in following the 21-day process. In his book *Spirituelles Heilen und Schulmedizin* (Spiritual healing and conventional medicine) he has given impressive expression to his own concept of life, his image of the human being and the world and his trust in the reality of the spirit. That such physicians exist and hold responsible medical positions – he is head of public psychiatric services in the Baselland Canton of Switzerland – is without any doubt exceedingly important for the future of medical science as a whole.

In his introduction to his own book he also hits the nail on the head as far as our present work is concerned in that he writes of a 'second awakening of science'. He argues in favour of a fundamental scientific attitude that does not allow itself to be restricted by scientific dogmas and materialistic doctrines but regards spiritual experiences and unusual phenomena as a call to bring about a change of paradigm. His whole book is interlaced with the basic idea that in reality there is no such thing as a rigid separation between matter and spirit. In this sense modern physics has already developed entirely new models that build bridges to a 'holistic view of the world'. For example he tells of experiments proving that prayer is effective in healing the sick, although the design of the experiment in such situations is always a matter for discussion.

The subject of receiving nourishment from light is only touched on in his book because he is concerned fundamentally with something far more all-encompassing, namely a new kind of science integrating the spiritual and wider dimension of the divine into our modern life with its corresponding effects in all branches of science, as was pioneered by Rudolf Steiner almost one hundred years ago through the spiritual science he referred to as anthroposophy. Bösch mentions Steiner and his work several times in his book.

In the section on observation and research in connection with the phenomenon of being nourished by light he writes:

> It is an important phenomenon that should not be pushed underground. This would only increase the dangers that do exist, as is shown by some deaths. This process of being nourished by light should be observed and researched under medical supervision with the involvement of the healing professions so that reliable information may soon be gained. A clinic devoted to the methods used by healers would be the right place to conduct such a project...*

Bösch's book concludes with a call to widen research into spiritual themes and questions: 'Spirituality in research would provide a wonderful interdisciplinary theme that would fill the lecture halls to bursting.' So what prevents this happening? In Bösch's opinion the time is ripe and the public would welcome such work, especially in the medical field. The main obstacle, he maintains, is the understanding of scientists and medical people who confuse 'objectivity' with materialism. 'They believe they must exclude consciousness from their research and view of the world in order to get closer to the truth; they fail to realize that the exclusion of consciousness has nothing to do with "objectivity" but instead causes them to drift ever further away from the healing truth.'

---

* Bösch, 2002.

6

Living without food yesterday and today

A brief historical survey and initial thoughts towards a scientific explanation *by Stephen Janetzko*

The phenomenon of living without food in all its many variations was being talked about long before Jasmuheen published her book. Early in the twentieth century Dr Karl Graninger, a physician in Graz, Austria, documented some 40 unusual cases of people who lived without eating for varying lengths of time. He was surprised by the fact that during the war people evidently reacted differently to having neither solid nor liquid nourishment. Some died of starvation while the health of others blossomed.

The best-known cases of living without food in Germany are those of Maria Furtner and Therese of Konnersreuth. Maria Furtner (1821–1884) was known in the upper Bavarian district of Rosenheim as 'the water drinker of Frasdorf'. For '52 years this peasant woman ingested nothing but water', a fact which is even immortalized on her gravestone. Therese Neumann (1898–1962) from Konnersreuth in Bavaria, another strictly Catholic peasant woman, consumed nothing but water for almost 40 years – from 1922 one or two spoonfuls a day, and from 1927 not even that – and the daily wafer at Holy Communion. According to some witnesses, even the wafer dematerialized on her tongue, so that no physical substance at all remained to be digested. So in effect she lived for 35 years without any kind of food.

The cases reported by Graninger and others had a number of traits in common: they were all pious and very sensitive individuals who were only conscious of their unusual destiny to a limited extent. Dr Albert A. Bartel, who carried on Graninger's work, said in addition that in most cases the circumstances which had led to the cessation of taking nourishment had pathological aspects: 'When young all of them had suffered from bone-marrow damage, i.e. in the blood-producing part of the body.' 'None of them suffered the nightmare of fearing death from starvation; the transitions to not eating were entirely painless.'

Paramahansa Yogananda, the well-known Indian master who had also visited Therese Neumann, reported on the story of an Indian woman, Giri Bala. At the time of his visit she had neither eaten nor drunk anything for 56 years. From childhood she had been noticed for her excessive greed, but then, having been criticized by her mother-in-law several times, she one day suddenly replied: 'I will soon show you that I shall take no more nourishment as long as I live.' And her prayers in this matter were indeed granted.

> 'It may be that all human beings receive 30 per cent of their nourishment from light, only in the normal run of things we are not aware of this.'*

But until Jasmuheen came along no one had felt called upon to 'live publicly' without ordinary food. Giri Bala said in this respect: 'The peasants would not thank me if I were to teach many people to live without food, for then the luscious fruits would lie rotting on the ground. It seems that want, famine and diseases are intended to be the scourges of our karma so that finally we may be helped to understand the true meaning of life.'

---

*This and all unattributed quotations in boxes by Michael Werner.

Apart from Jasmuheen and those who follow her in varying degrees there are today many cases of short-term abstention from food and drink. Nutrition adviser Roland Possin told me of his travels in South Dakota where the Lakota Indians, for example, undertake a four-day 'vision journey'. Many tribes abstain from food during such a journey, but the Lakota in addition abstain from any kind of fluid as well. In his book *Indianische Heilgeheimnisse*, Gerhard Buzzi, another expert on the Lakota, wrote: 'The vision-seeker was painted white and was accompanied by an experienced medicine man who prayed for him at the foot of the hill. For the next four days the seeker was alone – without food or drink, sunk in prayer with his pipe.'

So how can long periods of abstention from food be explained? At the spiritual level it sounds simple: Those who live on light derive their nourishment directly from the ether. Bartel* quotes A. von der Alz: 'It is assumed that all phenomena originate in an archetypal force, also called psi, and that in exceptional cases there are individuals who are linked with this force from which they are able to draw the energy which others have to derive from food.'

> 'Yet biophysicists today confirm that electro-magnetic radiation accounts for three quarters of the energy supplied and given off in humans and that quantitatively the acquisition of energy via food plays only a small part.'†

Bartel considers all former cases to be biochemically a kind of 'human plant': 'On account of some damage to the blood-generating organs, inediates [a person who doesn't eat] have coincidentally become a kind of human plant, whereby the

---

* 1976.
† Warnke, 1997, quoted by Bösch.

biochemical mechanism through which vital energy is created is made possible "at first-hand", i.e. by means of assimilation of carbon dioxide.' The open question is whether this condition can be brought into play deliberately without there being a pathological situation.

Professor Dr Georg Merkl recently suggested an interesting explanation for the ability to live without food: He has discovered that the energy-intensive process by means of which cells acquire adenosindiphosphate from adenosintriphosphate – an energy producing process that takes place primarily in the mitochondria, the 'power stations' of the cells – can be bypassed by a change in the conductivity of proteins: 'If all our proteins were to be super-conductive (i.e. possessed unlimited conductivity), then, with the help of this genetic material we would be able to bypass metabolic energy production and would only need to eat for pleasure rather than out of necessity.'

Professor Fritz-Albert Popp, biophoton expert from Kaiserslautern, Germany, has written in this connection:

I believe that in principle we do live on light. For example natural sugar is an excellent reservoir of light. The be all and end all is probably therefore the light-quality of our food. Personally I do not see any need to stop eating, but it seems to me to be not impossible. It would be good to study this further, since one frequently hears tales about it.*

In other words it would be a good thing to gain more scientific certainty about receiving nourishment through light and abstaining from food. Not only are individuals needed who are prepared to pass on their own experiences and, if the occasion arises, to subject themselves to regular scientific studies, but also

---

* Quoted in Janetzko, 1996.

courageous researchers who feel called upon to undertake such studies. There are also plans to set up the relevant training for interested therapists and medics so that continuous medical supervision can be provided for anyone wishing to embark on the process of receiving nourishment through light. (Christopher Schneider, govind@web.de)*

---

* Source: *ELRAANIS, Magazin für Lichtnahrung, Lichtarbeit und Spiritualität,* No. 3, Berlin 1998.

7

Historical and current examples

by Thomas Stöckli

As already explained, what interests us today is not whether some saint or yogi is able to experience things like living on light but whether there are natural forces that can work in ordinary human beings, a discovery which would provide a fundamental expansion of our scientific horizons. Historical examples not only throw light on the current phenomenon of living on light; they may also lead to a questioning of our present ideas or even to a complete re-thinking of them.

> 'It is an etheric energy that surrounds me and everything else; and once we have tapped it, it flows continuously. For the sake of simplicity we call it "nourishment from light", but it is not merely the effects of physical light that are meant. Rather it describes the totality of energies that surround us, which are also termed the "etheric forces".'

An Indian fakir as a 'challenge to science'

Here is a topical example recently discussed throughout the European media: Prahlad Jani, an Indian fakir aged 76, claims that he has neither eaten nor drunk anything for 65 years, thus disconcerting an unbelieving medical team. According to *The Hindustan Times* the deputy director of the hospital where the fakir was under observation stated: 'For ten days he has taken neither food nor drink, nor has he passed any urine or motions.' He was, however, physically and mentally fully fit and, according to one of his 'disciples', had never been ill. Another physician added that there was no explanation for this phenomenon, and that perhaps there was 'something divine' about it.

> *'The only precondition for being nourished by light is to have trust in it.'*

The report in the paper continued by stating that Jani, who normally lived near a temple in the Western Indian state of Gujarat, attributed his capability to a gift from the goddess Amba Mata. According to him, there had been a hole in his palate since he was a child out of which flowed a liquid which took the place of having to eat or drink. The medical team had confirmed that liquid flowed from a hole in his palate but had been unable to analyze it.

The BBC reported that Jani had been under constant CCTV surveillance during his stay in the hospital in Ahmedabad. In order to assist the doctors in monitoring him, Jani had also agreed to go without having a bath. 100 ml water daily – about half a glass – had been allowed for rinsing his mouth. The amount was measured again after he spat it out in order to ensure that he had not drunk any of it.

This very thin man with a long, snow-white beard who always wore red robes in honour of Amba Mata was, said the deputy director of the hospital, a 'challenge to science'. All the medical tests showed perfectly normal results. The doctors also said that while he was in the hospital urine appeared to form in his bladder and then be reabsorbed by the bladder wall.

Source: dpa-report of 26 November 2003 in the journal *Der Stern*.

Paramahansa Yogananda's encounter with Therese of Konnersreuth

There appears to be a not insignificant connection between these phenomena and the spiritual, indeed also the religious life, meaning an inner piety regardless of any adherence to a particular confession. We therefore include here the description of the encounter between Paramahansa Yogananda, as a representative of eastern spirituality, with the Christian mystic Therese Neumann who belonged to the Catholic faith and its Church:*

... for I wanted to make a pilgrimage to Bavaria. This would be my only chance, I felt, to visit the great Catholic mystic, Therese Neumann of Konnersreuth. Years earlier I had read an amazing account of Therese. Information given in the article was as follows:

(1) Therese, born on Good Friday in 1898, was injured in an accident at the age of twenty; she became blind and paralyzed.

(2) She miraculously regained her sight in 1923 through prayers to St Thérèse of Lisieux, 'The Little Flower'. Later Therese Neumann's limbs were instantaneously healed.

(3) From 1923 onward, Therese has abstained completely from food and drink, except for the daily swallowing of one small consecrated wafer.†

(4) The stigmata, sacred wounds of Christ, appeared in 1926 on Therese's head, breast, hands, and feet. Every Friday she experiences the Passion of Christ, suffering in her own body all his historic agonies. (Since the war years, Therese has not

---

* Quoted by kind permission of Self-Realization Fellowship.

† Self-Realization Fellowship does not endorse or recommend experimenting with reducing or eliminating consumption of food or water, without the guidance of a qualified health professional.

experienced the Passion every Friday but only on certain holy days of the year.)

(5) Knowing ordinarily only the simple German of her village, during her Friday trances Therese utters phrases which scholars have identified as ancient Aramaic. At appropriate times in her vision, she speaks Hebrew or Greek.

(6) By ecclesiastical permission, Therese has several times been under close scientific observation. Dr Fritz Gerlich, editor of a Protestant German newspaper, went to Konnersreuth to 'expose the Catholic fraud', but ended up by reverently writing her biography...

The following morning our party motored to the quiet town of Eichstätt. Dr Wutz greeted us cordially at his home: 'Yes, Therese is here.' He sent her word of the visitors. A messenger soon appeared with her reply: 'Though the bishop has asked me to see no one without his permission, I will receive the man of God from India.' Deeply touched at these words, I followed Dr Wutz upstairs to the sitting room. Therese entered immediately, radiating an aura of peace and joy. She wore a black gown and spotless white head-dress. Although her age was thirty-seven at this time, she seemed much younger; possessing indeed a childlike freshness and charm. Healthy, well-formed, rosy-cheeked, and cheerful, this is the saint who does not eat! Therese greeted me with a very gentle handshaking. We beamed in silent communion, each knowing the other to be a lover of God.

Dr Wutz kindly offered to serve as interpreter. As we seated ourselves, I noticed that Therese was glancing at me with naive curiosity; evidently Hindus had been rare in Bavaria.

'Don't you eat anything?' I wanted to hear the answer from her own lips.

'No, except a Host at six o'clock each morning.'

'How large is the Host?'

'It is paper-thin, the size of a small coin.' She added, 'I take it for sacramental reasons; if it is unconsecrated, I am unable to swallow it.'

'Certainly you could not have lived on that, for twelve whole years?'

'I live by God's light.' How simple her reply, how Einsteinian!

'I see you realize that energy flows to your body from the ether, sun, and air.'

A swift smile broke over her face. 'I am so happy to know you understand how I live.'

'Your sacred life is a daily demonstration of the truth uttered by Christ: Man shall not live by bread alone, but by every word that proceeds out of the mouth of God.'*

Again she showed joy at my explanation. 'It is indeed so. One of the reasons I am here on earth today is to prove that man can live by God's invisible light, and not by food only.'

'Can you teach others how to live without food?' She appeared a trifle shocked. 'I cannot do that; God does not wish it.'

As my gaze fell on her strong, graceful hands, Therese showed me a square, freshly healed wound on the back of each hand. On the palm of each hand, she pointed out a smaller, crescent-shaped wound, freshly healed. Each wound went straight through the hand. The sight brought to me a distinct recollection of the large square iron nails with crescent-tipped ends that are still used in the East but that I do not recall having seen in the West.

The saint told me something of her weekly trances. 'As a helpless onlooker, I observe the whole Passion of Christ.' Each week, from Thursday midnight until Friday afternoon at one o'clock, her wounds open and bleed; she loses ten pounds of her ordinary 121-pound weight. Suffering intensely in her sympa-

---

* Matthew 4,4.

thetic love, Therese yet looks forward joyously to these weekly visions of her Lord.

I realized at once that her life is intended by God to reassure all Christians of the historical authenticity of Jesus' life and crucifixion as recorded in the New Testament, and to display dramatically the ever living bond between the Galilean Master and his devotees.

Professor Wutz related some of his experiences with the saint. 'A group of us, including Therese, often travel for days on sightseeing trips in Germany,' he told me. 'It is a striking contrast – Therese eats nothing; the rest of us have three meals a day. She remains fresh as a rose, untouched by fatigue. Whenever the rest of us get hungry and look for wayside inns, Therese laughs merrily.'

The professor added some interesting physiological details: 'Because Therese takes no food, her stomach has shrunk. She has no excretions, but her perspiration glands function; her skin is always soft and firm.'

Therese Neumann died on 18 September 1962 in Konnersreuth.*

On the phenomenon of living without food or drink in the case of Therese Neumann

Living for years without food or drink is a frequent though not consistent accompaniment to stigmatization.

'As a scientist with considerable insight into modern medicine I have always been highly interested in the question: What is going on here?'

In the case of Therese of Konnersreuth the phenomenon of living without food or drink developed in stages. From Christmas

* Yogananda, 1993.

1922 onwards she took only liquids; then, from the festival of Christ's Transfiguration on 6 August 1926, 6 to 8 drops of water on a spoon to help swallow the sacred host. From September 1927 even this small amount of water was omitted.* However, it was evident that she could only survive if she received Holy Communion daily. If more than one day passed since the previous Communion she fell into a state of weakness that almost amounted to fainting from which she could only be roused by receiving the Eucharist once more. Among others, Chaplain Fahsel described this as follows: 'One first notices a clear increase in bodily strength. Beforehand she was often in a pitiable state of weakness ... Her face was small and hollow-cheeked. Dark rings surrounded her eyes. She could barely take her seat on her chair behind the altar. After her Communion all that disappears'.

> 'There is a clear experience of being nourished when one lives on light.'

Words spoken by Christ also refer to this replacement of natural by spiritual food: 'Moses gave you not that bread from heaven; but my Father gives you the true bread from heaven ... I am the living bread which came down from heaven ... And the bread that I will give is my flesh, which I will give for the life of the world ... For my flesh is meat indeed ...'.†

In view of the publicly expressed doubts as to Therese's abstention from food, the Bishop of Regensburg, Antonius von Henle, asked for medical confirmation of the phenomenon in 1927. Therese and then also her father agreed to an investigation from 14 to 28 July 1927 which consisted of a round-the-clock observation under medical supervision. Professor Ewald

---

* Teodorowicz.

† John 6,32; 6,51; 6,55.

and the episcopal office of Regensburg confirmed the result, which was that Therese did indeed abstain from all food.

> 'Today, scientists whose training has been cast in the traditional mould still feel annoyed and provoked by cases in which food, and especially liquids, have been refused for long periods.' (Jakob Bösch)

When discussion of Therese's abstention from nourishment again came into the public eye during the National Socialist period in Germany, the Cathedral Chapter of Regensburg insisted on a new investigation in 1936, this time in hospital, of her abstention from nourishment and her general state of health. Therese once again agreed. However, in view of demands from the National Socialist public that Therese should be incarcerated in a psychiatric clinic, her father feared for his daughter's safety if such an investigation were to be carried out. Since among others Professor Lechner, Eichstätt, as well as Cardinals Konrad von Preysing, Berlin, and Michael Faulhaber, Munich, were also warning against putting her in hospital, and especially as it had become known that 'undesirable elements' had lost their lives in hospital in mysterious circumstances or simply disappeared, he refused to give permission.

In 1940 another opportunity arose for Therese to be observed with a view to confirming her abstention from nourishment: 'From 7 to 13 July Therese lay semi-paralyzed in the Wutz household at Eichstätt after a stroke and was entirely dependent on help from others. Bishop Michael Rackl ordered that she be kept under strict observation for that period'.*

Statements on oath made by all the participants in the observation and investigation commission, including the physicians and university professors involved and also other wit-

---

* Steiner, J., 1988, p. 28.

nesses, prove Therese's complete abstention from food. This is also confirmed by all her relatives and other persons who had the opportunity to observe those around her and her own behaviour.

> 'Eating at table is a more coarse form of taking nourishment; respiration and sense perception – meaning an exchange which is like breathing with the senses – is a more subtle form of the same.'

At Eichstätt on 15 January 1953 Therese made the following declaration under oath regarding her abstention from nourishment:*

1. Although I cannot give the exact date, the reduction of food intake began during my illness after the accident in 1918, thus around 1918/19.

2. I have lived entirely without nourishment and with no desire for food or drink since Christmas 1926. From Christmas 1926 to September 1927 I partook of the Holy Body at Communion with a small spoonful of water. Since then this, too, has ceased. Since 6 August 1926 I have felt utter aversion and disgust with regard to food.

3. For a while I tried to take food in liquid form. However, I vomited it all (with retching) and therefore abandoned the attempt. Since giving up these efforts I have felt much better, as the retching occasioned by them and the heart problems that resulted have disappeared. From Christmas 1922 until today I have experienced the greatest difficulty in swallowing (when taking Holy Communion in its usual form).

4. ... I am convinced and know that I live on the sacramental Saviour who remains within me ... until shortly before the next Communion. Once the Sacramental Body dissolves I feel weak

---

* Steiner, J., 1977, p. 287.

and have a strong physical and mental longing for Holy Communion.

Source: www.thereseneumann.de

Are there still such phenomena today?

Therese Neumann was an example from the past, but what is the situation today in relation to such phenomena? In connection with mystical or religious experiences are there examples now of individuals who live without physical nourishment?

> *One cannot help suspecting that the real reason for the protests by both media and medical experts with regard to living on light boils down to the fact that such a way of life does not conform to prevailing views about the world.* (Jakob Bösch)

While working on this book we heard about another case, and Michael Werner was able to meet the person who does not at this point wish to speak publicly about herself. This woman works as a secretary and architect. During Easter Week in 2004 the stigmata manifested. According to those who know her these have remained virtually unchanged since then. As a result of the stigmata appearing her whole physical organism has been transformed. She has become more sensitive in her sense perceptions and profound changes have taken place in the way she receives nourishment. She stresses that this has come about not as the result of ascetic living but is the result of a bodily transformation. Her complete abstention from nourishment has caused neither loss of weight nor any other curtailments or physical complaints. The situation is rather that in its changed condition her body rejects any kind of earthly food. She can tolerate only small amounts of water.

This example shows that living without physical food can

occur as an accompaniment to something far greater. One can assume that in this case as also with Michael Werner the source from which the nourishment through light emanates is the being who says of himself: 'I am the light of the world.' The paths and also the initial motivations, however, are different. For the woman we have just described it was a religious experience that was the cause and starting point. Michael Werner, on the other hand, was searching for something through science and he made a conscious decision to try out a different way of receiving nourishment. Nevertheless, it seems that the two paths are related in some way, since Michael Werner also maintains that it is only possible where there is a real and profound trust in the spiritual world.

Nicholas von der Flüe

Looking back further in time we find that more than half a millennium ago Nicholas von der Flüe, the famous monk, was disturbing his contemporaries, provoking and upsetting their view of the world by surviving on no food at all.

> 'One aspect of this whole affair impressed me almost more than anything else: that in our seemingly so enlightened world of science, willingness to test and question basic concepts has if anything decreased but certainly not increased since the time of Galileo.' (Jakob Bösch)

Nicholas was born in 1417 on the Flüeli at Melchtal in the Swiss canton of Unterwalden. He was married to Dorothea with whom he had 10 children, five girls and five boys. In his fiftieth year, after a secular career as a farmer, soldier, judge and advocate, he withdrew from all personal and social obligations and went to live as a hermit in the valley of the Ranft near Melchtal, not far from his former home. As has been proved, he then lived for the following 20 years without taking any nourishment at all. He died aged 70 on his birthday, 21 March 1487, having by then come to be called Brother Klaus, the widely-known counsellor and wise man.

Johannes Hemleben, biologist and priest of the Christian Community, has summarized his ideas on the subject of nutrition and nourishment in a chapter of his book *Niklaus von Flüe*. His thoughts on the phenomenon of living without physical food are most revealing and we here quote at length from that chapter:

> The main difficulty we have today in understanding the fact that Brother Klaus lived without physical nourishment stems from what we are told by the science of nutritional physiology. This has now made great strides and gained insights into objective facts which cannot be doubted. However, they refer almost without exception to the first part of the nourishment process, the intake of substances, but not to the transmutation of substances. So we must turn our attention to the fundamental basis of human existence.
>
> From the biological point of view the human being is to a large extent a parasite on nature. He renders his physical existence possible by destroying his environment and recreating within himself what he has destroyed, shaping it to suit his own requirements. Settlements and streets, dwellings and clothes can only be created by breaking nature down and then reforming it to fit in with human purposes. And this basic law applies most especially to food. Salt, plants and animals are taken from nature, planted and harvested, cared for and guarded in flocks, always – as far as food is concerned – for the sole purpose of one day being annihilated and then incorporated. The initial rough breaking down or killing is usually followed by more refined processes of cutting up, grating and so on. Fire is used for

cooking to help make the food more palatable. Knives and forks are then used by civilized people for further mashing and chopping of nature's gifts, with only fruit needing nothing but the fingers.

The mouth and teeth form the boundary between 'outside' and 'inside'. This is where the nourishment process as such begins. Beyond the lips, the teeth continue the cutting, tearing and mashing, a purely physical process that serves further to destroy the natural substances before they are taken in by the organism. Having thus far been in contact only with the senses of touch, sight and smell, the food now enters the realm of the sense of taste through the mouth, the tongue and the palate. Here it is further dissolved by being mixed with saliva.

Strictly speaking, this is a process involving both body and soul which, expressed through tasting, also has a chemical component. Saliva contains the enzyme ptyalin which attacks especially all carbohydrates such as the starch found in bread, and takes them further into a process of disintegration and being split up. For a brief moment a healthy person can still feel, but not taste, how the chyme disappears down his throat. But from the end of the gullet onwards the eater will usually lose all awareness of the food. Only if something is wrong will pain draw attention to a process that normally runs its course without any further conscious contribution by the individual. Not until it comes to excretion will this totally unconscious process re-enter consciousness and require further action.

However, the ongoing procedure of being nourished, which takes place in bodily processes of which one is not aware, is all the more astonishing. Following on from receiving nourishment that involves external breaking-down and physical destruction, the organism continues the disintegration by chemical means. Let us mention only the most important stages of digestion known to us today. As soon as the chyme reaches the stomach it is flooded with the enzyme pepsin to continue with the further destruction of the food which the organism still treats as a foreign body. Pepsin dissolves the original composition of the proteins and splits these into peptons. On its way from stomach to intestines the food reaches the pancreas in the region of the duodenum which in turn begins to secrete the digestive enzyme trypsin. This continues the chemical process of dissolution, dissolving all still existing proteins from the food so that what remains is a homogeneous, viscous substance from which all traces of its origins have been eliminated. All that remains after the destruction of the carbohydrates and the proteins is the fat which has been eaten. This passes relatively unscathed through the regions where ptyalin and pepsin are active and is only broken down into glycerine and fatty acids by the enzyme lipase from the pancreas and bile. Some of the fat remains untouched by any of the digestive processes and is found relatively unchanged in the intestines. If it is not used up (to provide heat) or excreted, it can be stored in the body and thus – as a foreign substance – lead to disease.

We see that the process described very briefly here of receiving nourishment via the hand, the mouth and down to the intestines is from beginning to end governed by the principle of destroying and dissolving the food. From the point of view of the human body the process of taking in food is one of defence by the organism against the invading foreign substances. Ptyalin, pepsin, trypsin and lipase are an important part of the defence system whose task it is to divest foreign substances as far as possible of their original forces. This process of destruction in receiving nourishment has for the most part been made comprehensible by modern physiology. Radioactive and other methods have also enabled scientists to prove, in the living organism beyond the walls of the intestines, the presence of ingested substances in the blood, lymph and bones etc. But science has as yet failed to discover how the substances passing from the mouth to the intestines while being entirely divested of their substantial nature reappear on the other side of the intestinal wall in the various organs of the body not as bread, meat, drink and so on but as the flesh and blood of a living human being. In other words, the destruction of food and drink, of bread and wine, is observable and comprehensible. But we are still almost completely ignorant as to how food and drink, bread and wine become the body and blood of a living, individual human being.

Readers who have followed the argument thus far may now be taken aback when they realize that we have unexpectedly entered into the very centre of sacramental theology. The mystery of the sacrament at the altar is for its part also founded on the transmutation of bread and wine, but now into a 'higher' form of existence which in its religious context is known as 'the body and blood of Christ'. Is it not remarkable that the mystery of natural nourishment rests on the existential transmutation of food and drink into the body and blood of a natural human being? *As we have seen, this takes place for the most part in metabolic processes of which the human being is unaware. The mystery of this transmutation is brought about by the principle of nature which works within the human being without his being aware of it.*

Nicholas von der Flüe was profoundly associated with the sacrament at the Christian altar in its medieval form, and through it he experienced being given the most essential assistance in leading his life. This sacrament has taken the transmutation of bread (food) and wine (drink), that in nature occurs in the unconscious depths of the body's life, and raised it up into the light where it can be seen. Transubstantiation on the altar takes place before the eyes of the congregation not as a natural process but through the power of the priestly mandate aided by the spiritual help of a believing community. Here the substances of nature are transmuted in a sphere that leads to one which lies beyond nature. It is the world of the Risen One. The visible bread and the visible wine become bearers of the supersensible body and blood of Christ. In the language of theology: The kingdom of God, which is not of this world, appears in this world and transmutes it to a higher plane of existence. Aided by his prayerful life Nicholas von der Flüe shared in this power of transformation in more than the ordinary way.

It goes without saying that we should not allow ourselves to belabour this comparison and make of it an absolute, thus denying the difference between physiological transmutation and sacramental transubstantiation. In physiological transmutation the physical substances which begin by being visible are destroyed to the extent of becoming unrecognizable, only to become visible again as the substantiality of body and blood in the living organism. In the sacrament at the altar the bread and wine remain visible even after the transubstantiation and are then 'incorporated' into human beings through the communion. The body and blood of Christ, meanwhile, remain invisible. The mystery of transubstantiation rests on the invisible transformation of visible substances.

Whereas ordinary nourishment, i.e. the transmutation of food-stuffs, takes place invisibly within the organism, the sacrament at the altar takes place by invisible means in full view of the congregation. Both involve the attainment of a higher stage of existence.

Ordinary nourishment is subject to entirely natural laws. Everything that has been said here about the physiological processes involved is valid in principle both for human beings and the higher animals, and in a variety of other forms also for all living creatures. Transubstantiation at the altar, however, takes place only if human beings will it and behave and act accordingly during the service. In the days when a pious yet knowing relationship with the body and blood of Christ was still felt and cultivated, people knew that the sacrament involved not the 'natural' forces of the human being but 'supernatural' forces which streamed towards them from another sphere of existence when they sought them in an appropriate way.

This presupposes that the seeker finds a way of relating to what is known in Christianity as the *working* of grace. Human beings can subject nature to their will, but the power of the Risen One cannot be touched by it; *they can only receive grace if they have learned to be humble and modest. This is what was meant by medieval Christian theologians when they said: One can know nature, but one must believe in what is above nature, in the supernatural.*

As the modern age dawned this duality of mental life became increasingly problematical. Modern individuals wanted and still want to be able to think and know about the content of their religious beliefs. This problem did not exist for Nicholas von der Flüe. He was one of the few in his day who not only received with piety the working of the sacrament at the altar but also, though he was not a priest, experienced the transubstantiation in full consciousness again and again. For him his belief was conscious experience and this experience in turn was living knowledge. Just as a person with healthy eyes cannot doubt the existence of the sun, so did Brother Klaus not doubt the higher reality of the body and blood of Christ upon the altar ... Although he saw a good deal that was not right in his church, this would never have been a reason for him to turn away from it. However worthy or unworthy different priests might be, the validity of the priesthood and the sacrament were for him beyond all doubt. Indeed, how could he have doubted a happening the higher reality of which he was ever and again able to experience? Just as ordinary people need their daily food as a matter of course, so through prayer and the sacrament at the altar did Nicholas von der Flüe draw strength as a matter of course for his whole being right down into his physical body.

It is only natural for people to disagree about such things. Throughout the 20 years of his total abstinence from food Brother Klaus lived in the experience of a supersensible reality. Both then and now, those who have no access to an experience of this sphere are likely to doubt that he never ate food. But they are like a person born blind who refuses to let a sighted person tell them about colours. In such situations discussion is likely to prove fruitless. But the words of Brother Klaus are beyond discussion: Upon contemplating the separation of Christ's soul from his body in the renewal of the Passion, he felt his heart filled with an indescribable tenderness so refreshing that it became easy for him to do without ordinary human food.*

---

* Hemleben, 1977.

8

Analytical psychology as a helpful source of ideas and suggestions

by Thomas Stockli

In addition to modern physics and Rudolf Steiner's spiritual science, valuable aids to understanding the process of living on light can also be gained from C. G. Jung's analytical psychology. Perhaps collaboration between these three ways of thinking will be needed in developing models that can explain the phenomenon of drawing nourishment from light. It is also our hope that science will be spurred on to take a further step into the twenty-first century by its present inability to explain such phenomena.

In his book *Tachyonen, Orgonenergie, Skalarwellen. Feinstoffliche Felder zwischen Mythos und Wissenschaft* ('Tachyons, Orgone energy, Scalar waves, Subtle fields, Between Myth and Science'), Marco Bischof has provided some very interesting suggestions which we cite below:

The power of the imagination and the physical-material world

The power of imagination is the 'formative force' talked of by Blumenbach and Steiner; in the language of alchemy it is called 'God's imagination' as stated by C. G. Jung in his work *Psychology and Alchemy*. An alchemical treatise states: 'What God imagines comes about in reality, but what the soul imagines is merely something mental.' This appears to correspond exactly to the superficial prejudice which maintains that everything seen in mental images 'is merely fantasy' and imaginary, whereas in reality such images contain the recipe for effective imagination: Only when the imagining comes from our super-individual, inmost divine core is it a force that creates reality, but not when it stems merely from our individual psyche.

As C. G. Jung wrote in connection with alchemy, true imagination is far more than mere fantasy or wishful thinking. Imaginative processes 'take place in an intermediate sphere between matter and spirit, in a soul realm of subtle bodies that have both spiritual and material appearances, that are something like a body, a subtle *corpus* of a semi-spiritual nature'. Jung emphasizes that imagination is 'a force that can bring about change both in the soul realm and in the bodily realm'. It is also the 'power of divining', the power conceived of in the Middle Ages that manifested in the use of the divining rod ... Divining must be conceived of as a force with magical effect.

The etheric realm is that subtle dimension of reality in which there proceeds the divining, wishing and imagining of possibilities which is the preliminary stage of manifestation. It is the level of virtual reality where all potentially possible forms and events of which prototypical images are 'laid down in the world of archetypes' can 'work themselves through' and as it were try out their existence, but where it is not yet decided what form their ultimate manifestation will take. On this 'rehearsal stage of reality', forms and possibilities are tried out and in some cases rejected until the decision is made as to which shall become manifest. This decision is made by the self, by the inmost being, which is something which works not only in the individual human being but also in the inmost core of all the processes of reality.

According to the Shiite tradition of the 'Three-World-Doctrine' described by Henry Corbin, imagination is also the organ of perception for 'the world of the imaginal', the level of the etheric, but also the world of objects with the seven ordinary senses and the world of 'pure forms and intelligences' (archetypes) which are perceived with 'intellectual intuition'. According to Corbin, the world of the imaginal is 'less material than the physical world but more material than the world of the intellect. It is a world of subtle bodies, of spiritual bodies whose mode of existence is one of *being in abeyance* and which possess their own kind of materiality.' In my opinion, it is of the greatest importance for future scientific research into the subtle realm that traditional science points both to the nature of the subtle realm as containing the prephases of manifestion and also to the central significance of human consciousness and imagination as collaborating formative forces of this process.

C.G. Jung's Unus Mundus

A further scientific conception that throws significant light on the nature of the vacuum and the subtle realm is Carl Gustav Jung's *Unus Mundus*. This conception, which was subsequently interpreted and expanded by Jung's pupil Marie-Luise von Franz, arose from his collaboration with the physicist Wolfgang Pauli which is documented in their book *The Interpretation of Nature and the Psyche*. It provides the model which the two researchers hoped to apply to bringing quantum physics, analytical psychology and parapsychology closer to one another.

The idea of *Unus Mundus* rests on the assumption that the diversity of the empirical world is founded on a profound oneness. *Unus Mundus* is a uniform all-world background in which all opposites are still united, thus especially multiplicity and unity, psyche and matter. The concept originated in medieval Scholasticism where it denoted the potential archetypal world plan existing in the mind of God before creation began. This 'transcendent psycho-physical background' of our reality is the foundation both of the material world and the world of psyche and consciousness. It is 'as much physical as psychic and therefore neither of these but rather a third "something" which can only be intimated'. This uniform level of existence is a 'potential structure' that lies outside space and time but manifests sporadically in the consciousness while not being directly accessible to sensory perception . . .

Jung and von Franz also had something to say about the 'energy question': Psychic energy and physical energy, both of which originate in the *Unus Mundus* and are structured by the *Unus Mundus*, are an expression of the dynamic processes in the all-world background. Both are numerically structured. Von Franz wrote that the natural numbers are 'the typical, everywhere-repeated common pattern of movement of psychic and physical energy'. Jung considered that at the level of *Unus Mundus* not only did the psychic manifest 'a certain latent physical energy' and effectiveness, but that matter also possessed a latent psychic nature. According to Jung, this psychic energy consists of a certain 'physical intensity' which, if it were measurable, would manifest as something spread out and moving in space. Jung also considered it possible that psychic reality could extend to matter, especially in moments of synchronicity. He called for the establishment of a new branch of science which could research such phenomena.

9

Light and food – a glance into history

by Michael Werner

Many ancient cultures, especially in their creation stories, point to the important role light has played in the evolution of the earth. Western traditions too, with their roots in Biblical history, contain interesting hints about light, nourishment and food which are worth pondering. Some of those most worthy of consideration are cited here.

Ancient cultures

Both the *Rigvedas* and the *Samavedas* of ancient India begin with the words: 'Agni milet prohitam' ('I revere the fire'). The first word, from which all the rest follows, is 'agni', fire, the expression for light and heat, the beginning and source of creation. According to Zarathustra, the teacher and leader of ancient Persia, the world first developed out of the polarity of light and darkness with their representatives Ormuzd and Ahriman battling for power over human beings. Zarathustra's teachings call for his pupils to acknowledge the light and fight to overcome and redeem the darkness.

The old Germanic tradition, described so impressively for example in the *Edda*, also recognizes the significance of light. The death of Baldur, god of light, ushers in the time of darkness on the earth, the twilight of the gods. In a high-spirited game Hödur accidentally kills his brother Baldur because the dark and cunning god Loki has betrayed blind Hödur by treacherously handing him the fatal arrow of mistletoe which kills Baldur. The world of the gods is lost to men, and humanity can only find its way back to the light through its own initiative.

There are hints concerning the taking of nourishment even in the ancient Indian tradition. In the crucial portion of the Mahabharata Epic, the *Bhagavad Gita* or 'Song of the Lord', Arjuna, representative of humanity, is initiated into the divine secrets by the god Krishna on the battlefield shortly before the battle begins. On the subject of food he states that there is not much point in not eating since by itself this would not suffice as a way of achieving oneness with the divine: 'For the embodied being who does not feed on them the objects of sense disappear, except flavour; flavour fades too for the one who has seen the highest' (II, verse 59). He also says that only consecrated food should be eaten: 'The virtuous who eat the remainder of the sacrifice are released from all faults; the wicked who cook for the sake of themselves consume impurity' (III, verse 13). 'Others, who have put limits on their consumption of food, offer their inhalation into their inhalation. All these, who know what sacrifice is, have their imperfections obliterated by sacrifice' (IV, verse 30).*

The western tradition

Here the strongest conceptions of the creation and evolution of the world stem above all from the images of the Old Testament. Heaven and earth are created on the first day. The earth is without form and void. Then God's mighty word brings movement into creation: 'And God said, let there be light: and there was light. And God saw the light, that it was good: and God divided the light from the darkness' (Genesis 1, 1–4). We notice that the creation of the sun together with the moon and stars,

---

* *The Bhagavad Gita.*

which are for us inseparable from the phenomenon of light on the earth, only takes place on the fourth day. So one has to ask what is meant by the light created on the first day.

> 'It is quite simply a ubiquitous energy that is everywhere present, and one of the ways in which it reveals itself is in light. Light forms the boundary between the material and the immaterial. It also has those delicately contrasting qualities arising from its wave nature on the one hand and its particle nature on the other, its wave-particle duality. It functions at the boundary between the material and the spiritual, which is why "living on light" does after all remain the best way of describing it.'

The process of creation is brought up again in the New Testament, but here it is more abstract and less pictorial. In the prologue to the Gospel of John we read: 'In the beginning was the Word … In him was life; and the life was the light of men. And the light shines in the darkness; and the darkness comprehended it not' (John 1, 1–5). This last sentence reminds us of Zarathustra's requirement in the ancient Persian tradition to acknowledge the light and thus illumine and redeem the darkness. It also reminds us of the tragic Baldur tale in Germanic mythology which points to humanity's task that today still remains unresolved and unfinished. The god of light, Baldur, continues to wait for his redemption, and the crucified Christ for his brothers and sisters.

Food, too, is mentioned in the Biblical story of creation. On the sixth day God creates the human being and gives him 'herbs that bear seeds' and 'trees that bear fruit … which shall be for meat' (Genesis 1,29). The fall and expulsion from Paradise are punishment for yielding to the temptation of the cunning serpent and eating that which may not be eaten: the fruit of the tree of knowledge. So now the human being has to make his own provision for what he needs for life: Abel becomes the first shepherd and Cain the first tiller of the soil. The cultivation of physical food begins and becomes increasingly refined as time goes on.

'Our daily bread'

Light and food are also mentioned in the Moses story of the burning bush in which 'the angel of the Lord' appears, and in the 'bread' that falls from heaven as manna in conjunction with the challenge to believe and have trust because 'man does not live by bread only but by every word that proceeds out of the mouth of the Lord' (Deuteronomy 8,3). This is one of the first indications of an inexplicable, incomprehensible and thus miraculous provision of food. After his 40-day 'fast' in the desert, Christ uses these same words from the Old Testament when he rejects the devil's temptation to turn stones into bread. Later on this 'bread miracle' occurs several times but for other reasons and with different intentions: for example at the 'feeding of the five thousand' (Matthew 14, 19–20) when a multitude of five thousand are miraculously fed with only five loaves and two fishes.

In this connection it is worth looking more closely at the request for 'our daily bread' in the Lord's Prayer. Neil Douglas-Klotz (1992) points out that the common language at the time of Christ was Aramaic, which was spoken and understood by almost all the peoples of the Near East far beyond the boundaries of present-day Palestine. Therefore the 'original texts' of the Gospels written in Greek or Latin need to be read with care. The Aramaic language has a strong connection with nature and an integrated understanding of the world and all living creatures which is quite different from the dialectic and rational approach of Greek or, even more so, Latin. Douglas-Klotz demonstrates this using the Lord's Prayer and the Beatitudes as examples, providing the reader with a new and more comprehensive understanding of these texts. Thus, for example, the word *shem* as *shemaya* can mean 'heaven', as in the first line of the Lord's Prayer, or 'name' as in the second line, or, more generalized, 'light', 'sound' or 'experience'. Regarding the entreaty 'Give us this day our daily bread' (in Aramaic: *Hawvlan lachma d'sunkanan jaomana*) we have to remember that the Aramaic word *lachma* is correctly translated as 'bread'. But in addition the Aramaic word for 'bread' can also refer to any kind of food, even spiritual food, and may also mean 'sacred wisdom'. So in Aramaic the words for 'nourishment from light', 'nourishment from spirit' and 'nourishment from bread' intermingle with one another, which means that the distinctions which our language makes us draw cannot nor should be made in Aramaic.

It is in this sense that the significance of differentiating between material-physical well-water and 'living water' in the account of the meeting with the woman of Samaria becomes comprehensible (John 4, 1–34). And the same goes for the material-physical bread and the 'bread of life' when Christ says to his disciples: 'Your fathers ate manna in the desert and perished. This is the bread that comes from heaven so that the one who eats it shall not perish. Whoever eats my flesh and drinks my blood, he shall have eternal life.'

Finally, at the Last Supper the transubstantiation of bread and wine into the forces of the body and blood of Christ and thus into eternal life is shown as an example for all future times (Matthew 26, 17–30). Thus are the forces of darkness conquered or made conquerable, which allows Paul the Apostle to find the words of redemption: 'Death, where is your sting? Hell, where is your victory?'

The Eucharist as an explanatory model

Seen in the light of spiritual science, the Eucharist can be regarded as a model which gives us important insights into the phenomenon of nourishment that is both spiritual and physical. Conditioned, perhaps, by ecclesiastical traditions that are restrictive or dogmatic, we as modern scientists may simply be insufficiently open to the possibility of including this 'mystery' as a thesis in our considerations. Perhaps the 'resurrection corporeality' can work in a transforming way right down into an individual's physical constitution and bring about changes there through a form of 'nourishing communion' that can take place independently outside ecclesiastical tradition. Since they possess their own laws and ways of being effective, surely neither 'spirit' nor 'resurrection forces' can be determined by human beings.

Rudolf Frieling used Christian terminology to express what lies behind transubstantiation and communion:

> If Christ is accepted within, the process of metamorphosis gradually permeates the whole human being and finally reaches the depths of his body. 'Therefore, if any one is in Christ, he is a new creation' (*ktisis*, 2 Cor. 5,17). In becoming Christian, it is a matter of the whole human being experiencing a union, accepting an absolutely real influence into his own being; this is experienced in the Eucharist which has been celebrated in Christendom from the beginning (Acts 2, 46). In John's account of the Feeding of the Five Thousand, which seems like an anticipation of the mystery of the Eucharist just a year before Golgotha, the relationship of the Christian to Christ is expressed in the briefest way: 'He who eats me...' (John 6, 57). The unifying process begins in the spiritual region of the soul, yet the further it goes the deeper it invades the lower levels of the human being, till it finally reaches the body. The early Christians felt

vitally that through the bread and wine of the Eucharist they were connected with the Resurrection Body of Christ; the Communion was for them *pharmakon athanasias*, medicine for immortality (Letter of Ignatius to the Ephesians 20, 2).*

Light as such has always and everywhere been perceived and esteemed by human beings with much gratitude and veneration. In people's own experience of warmth and healing, in their view of nature and the growing and thriving of plants and animals, in their experience of the weather and the alternation between day and night, the importance of the sun's light was known to be the source of a higher creative power for thousands of years before science discovered photosynthesis and with it the transition from the non-organic and dead to the organic and living by means of the metamorphosis of carbon dioxide and oxygen into sugar and its related substances.

> 'We have known at the latest since the development of quantum theory that light and matter are different states of the same thing. And we have known since the discovery of photosynthesis that sunlight can produce starch, i.e. solid matter or foodstuffs, out of CO_2 and H_2O, though to this day this process is still not scientifically understood in every detail.' (Jakob Bösch)

For modern physics the phenomenon of 'light' remains a riddle that defies exact definition. This, too, is significant, since light stands like a guard and a messenger at the boundary between physics and metaphysics. Arthur Zajonc, professor of physics with a special interest in quantum physics has written in detail on this theme in his book *Catching the Light* in which he also looks at Rudolf Steiner's 'metaphysics of light' that shows

---

* Frieling, 1975.

the correlation between the natural world and the world of spirit and morality.*

We surely miss the point when we look on light and food as being alternative issues. One of the best answers to the question: 'Bread or light?' may be found in the well-known saying of the medieval mystic Angelus Silesius:

> It is not bread that feeds us.
> What feeds us in the bread
> is God's eternal word,
> is spirit and is life!

---

* Zajonc, 1993.

Conclusion

'*May the idea of what is pure, extended even to include the morsel of food in the mouth, become ever more filled with light.*' (J. W. von Goethe)

There is much upon which we may reflect in conclusion:

To find our way out of the materialistic cul-de-sac into which we have got ourselves we shall, in our time, be obliged to discover a new kind of inwardness, a religious life not bounded by doctrine, a true sense of how the world is manifested, a science that also embraces the spirit. Shaking us up by means of various events and phenomena, the spiritual world is endeavouring to extricate us from our ingrained habits of thought. Perhaps wonderment and reverence will be the starting point, but our critical faculties should not be disregarded.

'*All knowledge needs some kind of wonderment as the seed out of which it may grow.*' (Rudolf Steiner)

We do surely live in the midst of an ocean of life forces! Without realizing it we move in an 'etheric sea' like fishes in the ocean. The strength of our trust in this world of spirit, our openness towards nourishment received from spiritual powers, our search to find the good beings who are at home here – all this brings special forces into our world, forces that are not of this earth. It is not a matter of ceasing to eat; the important thing is not to shut ourselves off through materialistic ideas about nutrition or about how we take energy and life into ourselves. Is it perhaps possible that we have at our disposal an infinite reservoir of energy and life forces from which we are separated solely by our limited image of the world and of the human being? These forces need us to make space for them consciously and in freedom; they need us to invite them into the space within us and into the space all around us. They are the forces of living beings emanating from the source of the Primeval Being who overcame death and who 'will return in the clouds' (like a life-giving, nourishing rain), and who said of himself: 'I am the life!' (Heidenreich 1969; Stöckli 1991).

> Give us this day our daily spirit food
> You approach us in the bread,
> You draw near in water, air and light.
> Let us each day more clearly see
> How god's own force our body makes.
> With thanks we break it with our hands
> While knowingly our mouths may say:
> You approach us in the bread,
> You draw near in water, air and light.
> (Martin Rothe)

The time has come for us to expand and add to our image of the human being and the world, and for us radically to question present attitudes. Today's view of the world has grown histori-cally and it will continue to evolve. We can participate in this development. If this book has been able to give any impetus to the process, it will have fulfilled its purpose.

> Ecce homo
> Yes! I know whence I have come!
> Like a flame, insatiable,
> Glowing I myself devour.

All I receive is turned to light,
All I relinquish is carbon only:
Surely, sure I am a flame.
(Friedrich Nietzsche)

Afterword to the English edition

As we commenced work on the 2004 German edition of this book, planning for the first ever scientific investigation into receiving nourishment from light had just been put in train, and appeared to all those involved to be progressing nicely. It was our intention from the outset to include, as one of the main chapters, the results of some well-conducted research. But even as the study was progressing, with Michael Werner incarcerated at the clinic in Berne, and more recently during preliminary evaluation of the data, it became clear that interpretation and subsequent publication of the results in a scientific journal would be beset by more difficulties than had been expected.

In the main this can be explained by the fact that a number of 'ifs and buts' arose that left too wide a margin open to interpretation, chiefly on account of the test subject's unexpected weight loss which, in view of the understandably ticklish theme of 'nourishment without food', necessitated complicated discussions before scrupulously considered conclusions could be reached.

A further problem was that the responsible study directors have experienced great reluctance, which we fully understand and endorse, with regard to presenting such ambiguous results to a scientific community which is anyway very sceptical about, and in some cases downright hostile towards, phenomena like that of receiving nutrition from light.

Once we realized that considerably more delay would be unavoidable we therefore decided in the spring of 2004 to go ahead with the German-language edition of our book in which we would include a preliminary personal account of the study, while still entertaining hopes that a scientific publication was not too far away. As the months passed, however, we began to realize that work on publication of the study continued to be delayed, and to date (April 2007) its results remain unavailable for quotation or discussion. We have, however, recently been informed by the study directors responsible for publication that the manuscript has meanwhile been completed and that subject to some last-minute fine-tuning of certain formulations is about to be sent to the publishers of a suitable scientific journal.

Thus shortly before the first English-language edition of our book goes to press we find ourselves in an unsatisfactory situation rather like the one we experienced two years ago when bringing out the German edition.

However, we are happy to report that the media together with the German-speaking public have received the book very positively, realizing that the intention is not to cause a 'sensation' but to give pause for thought and show by example that there is still much in the world today that cannot yet be explained by science. They have been sensitive to the fact that the book has arisen from the work of individuals who are both critical and self-critical, who not only eschew dogmatism and are willing to live with many open questions, but who also wish to oppose any dogmatism whether it comes from the scientific fraternity or from spiritually-oriented or religious groupings. Indeed the media have almost without exception succeeded in bringing together contradictory opinions in an objective manner without in any way poking fun at the phenomenon or sidelining it by sensationalism. There has also been great demand for the book, necessitating several reprints of the German version. So all in all we are much encouraged.

Our conclusions

Our initial endeavours to bring the phenomenon to the attention of a wider public began in 2004, and we have now accepted that publication of the scientific evaluation is going to take quite a long time. The way the study was designed anyway means that evaluation will be muted, and we have also meanwhile reached certain critical conclusions about it ourselves.

We have been in contact with a number of institutes and also university professors, but there are as yet no plans for a new research project although a number of people have shown an interest. There will, however, be a follow-up project at the University of Prague in May 2007.

We do understand on the one hand that scientists have different priorities (mainstream projects that are more likely to earn them greater academic acclaim and attract more copious funding) and that universities, too, seek out projects that come with ready-made funding or will enhance their academic rating. Why should the scientific world want to cause raised eyebrows by getting involved in such a radical and 'problematical' exploration?

But on the other hand we have not ceased to hope that others will also find this topic very exciting and capable of yielding new insights that will not fail to attract the interest of an open-minded and enthusiastic scientific fraternity. Science is always enlivened by being confronted with new facts waiting to be critically investigated. The new models developed in consequence often yield epoch-making discoveries.

In fact leading universities keep pointing out that the time has come for a paradigm change. A few years ago global warming as a subject of research only interested a few NGOs like Greenpeace and some scientific outsiders, yet now it has become a reputation-enhancing scientific field in its own right. Is it not possible that in the field of 'human energy' the questions we have been discussing here might also in future become a respectable focus of research interest?

We believe that the phenomenon we have been describing calls for a paradigm change of this kind. But first it will be necessary to prove entirely objectively and critically that Michael Werner has indeed been and still is hale and hearty after living for a good many years without eating food. In doing this it will be important for the setting of the next study to be more bio-friendly in order to prevent or at least reduce the biological stresses mentioned on pages 156 and 157. Perhaps a study involving a 'metabolic chamber' could be devised, or an inter-faculty effort including the social sciences (in which PhD students might be employed in investigating individual cases). We can report that in the interim two gatherings have already taken place here in Switzerland, each with about 50 participants all of whom had carried out the 21-day process and many of whom are still living without any ordinary solid food. These people are all personally known to Michael Werner, a fact that is surprising in itself. Perhaps it could provide the background for some research with a sociological ingredient involving in-depth interviews that might yield more insights.

One academic noted the following in his review of the German edition of this book:

[What] can only be ignored with difficulty is the phenomenon itself, for it is crying out to be noticed. One wonders why mainstream science has paid so little attention to it, with offers to participate in studies being politely declined. There are two possibilities we can consider. Either Werner and his co-author

Stöckli are fraudsters or else they are drawing attention to a phenomenon of utmost importance. The first of these seems to me to be extremely unlikely, since it would be hard to find a scientist, especially one working in the pharmaceutical field, who would be willing to risk being unmasked as a fraudster. This being the case, note should be taken of the phenomenon so that we can begin a process of fundamental thought about the foundation on which our conception of science rests. As a tool for such a process, this book provides good documentation and plenty of material. (Harald Walach, Research Professor of Psychology, University of Northampton, and Director of the European Office of the Samueli Institute, in *Forschende Komplementärmedizin – Klassische Naturheilkunde*, 2005, 12:241–242.)

Let us bring this publication to a close with a call to scientists, wherever they may be working, to come to grips with this phenomenon with a view to setting up suitable case studies. As Michael Werner's example shows, there is no shortage of subjects who would be willing to participate.

Michael Werner and Thomas Stöckli
April 2007

APPENDIX

A number of references are made in this book to the scientist and philosopher Rudolf Steiner (1861–1925), in whose work both authors have an interest. It should be noted, however, that Steiner never spoke about the notion of living without food or 'living on light', and this practise has no explicit connections with his teaching or with the Anthroposophical Society he founded.

Steiner called his spiritual philosophy 'anthroposophy', meaning 'wisdom of the human being'. As a highly developed seer, he claimed to have direct knowledge and perception of spiritual dimensions, initiating a 'science of the spirit' that he hoped to make accessible to anyone willing to exercise unprejudiced thinking.

A true polymath, from his spiritual investigations Steiner provided suggestions for the renewal of many activities, including education (both general and special), agriculture, medicine, economics, architecture, science, philosophy, religion and the arts. Today there are thousands of schools, clinics, farms and other organizations involved in practical work based on his principles. His many published works feature his research into the spiritual nature of the human being, the evolution of the world and humanity, and methods of personal development.

Steiner wrote some 30 books and delivered over 6000 lectures across Europe, and in 1924 founded the General Anthroposophical Society, which today has branches throughout the world.

Bibliography

Aretin, Erwin Freiherr von: *Die Sühneseele von Konnersreuth*, Siegfried Hacker, Gröbenzell near Munich, n.d.

Arzt, Thomas et al (Ed.): *Unus Mundus – Kosmos und Sympathie*, Peter Lang, Frankfurt am Main 1992.

Balsekar, Ramesh S.: *Erleuchtende Gespräche*, Alf Lüchnow, Freiburg 1994.

Bartel, Albert A.: 'Sie wurden zu menschlichen Pflanzen. Überraschende Erklärung für das Phänomen der Nahrungslosigkeit' in: *Esotera* 11 (1976): 1020–1029.

The Bhagavad Gita, Oxford World Classics, Oxford 1994 (Trs. W. J. Johnson).

Bischof, Marco: *Tachyonen, Orgonenergie, Skalarwellen. Feinstoffliche Felder zwischen Mythos und Wissenschaft*, AT Verlag, Aarau 2002.

Bösch, Jakob: *Spirituelles Heilen und Schulmedizin*, Buchverlag Lokwort, Berne 2002.

Buzzi, Gerhard: *Indianische Heilgeheimnisse*, G. Lübbe Verlag, Bergisch Gladbach 1997.

Douglas-Klotz, Neil: *Das Vaterunser*, Knaur, Munich 1992.

Dürr, Hanns-Peter, Oesterreicher M.: *Wir erleben mehr als wir begreifen*, Verlag Herder, Freiburg i. Br., 2001.

Franz, Marie Louise von: *Zahl und Zeit*, Ernst Klett Verlag, Stuttgart 1970; 1988.

Frieling, Rudolf: *Christianity and Reincarnation*, Floris Books, Edinburgh 1977 (Trs. R. and M. Koehler).

Heidenreich, Alfred: *The Risen Christ and the Etheric Christ*, Rudolf Steiner Press, London 1969.

Hemleben, Johannes: *Niklaus von Flüe*, Verlag Huber, Frauenfeld 1977.

Jahn, R. G.: 'Information, Consciousness and Health', in: *Alternative Therapies* 2/3 (1996): 32–38.

Janetzko, Stephen: 'Nahrungslosigkeit gestern und heute. Ein historischer Kurzüberblick und erste wissenschaftliche Erklärungsversuche' in: *ELRAANIS – Magazin für Lichtnahrung, Lichtarbeit und Spiritualität*, 3 (1998): 60–61, Berlin 1998.

Janetzko, Stephen: 'Rohe Kost für feine Sinne' in: *esotera* 11 (1996): 54–57.

Jasmuheen: *Living on Light. The Source of Nourishment for the New Millennium*, 2nd edition, KOHA Publishing, Germany 1998.
(E-book version: *Pranic Nourishment. Nutrition for the New Millennium*, Self Empowerment Academy, Australia 2006.)

Jung, C. G.: *Collected Works of C. G. Jung*, Princeton University Press, Vols. 1–21, 1970–2000.

Lüpke, Geseko von: *Politik des Herzens*, Arun Verlag, Engeerda 2003.

Merkl, Georg: *Geflüster aus dem Kosmos*. Internet at:
http://ourworld.compuserve.com/homepages/Mengmann/
sumer3.htm.

Pauli, Wolfgang and Jung, C. G.: *Naturerklärung und Psyche*, Rascher Verlag, Zurich 1952.

Possin, Roland: *Die Stimme des Körpers. Ernährung im Einklang mit der inneren Führung*, Bastei-Lübbe, Bergisch Gladbach 1998.

Steiner, Johannes: *Therese Neumann von Konnersreuth. Ein Lebensbild nach authentischen Berichten, Tagebüchern und Dokumenten*, Schnell & Steiner, Munich/Zurich 1988.

Steiner, Johannes: *Visionen der Therese Neumann*, Schnell & Steiner, Munich/Zurich 1977.

Steiner, Rudolf: *Manifestations of Karma* (GA 120), Rudolf Steiner Press, London 1995, (Trs. H. Herrmann-Davey).

Steiner, Rudolf: *Agriculture* (GA 327), Bio-Dynamic Farming and Gardening Association Inc., Kimberton 1993 (Trs. C. Creeger and M. Gardner).

Steiner, Rudolf: *From Mammoths to Mediums* (GA 350), Rudolf Steiner Press, London 2000 (Trs. A. Meuss).

Stöckli, Thomas: 'Der Mensch lebt nicht nur vom Brot allein' in *Das Goetheanum*, 34/35(2002): 626.

Stöckli, Thomas: *Wege zur Christus-Erfahrung. Das Ätherische Christuswirken*, Verlag am Goetheanum, Dornach 1991.

Vandereycken, W. et al.: *Hungerkünstler, Fastenwunder, Magersucht*, dtv, Munich 1992.

Warnke U.: *Gehirn-Magie*, Popular Academic Verlag, Saarbrücken 1997.

Wegman, Ita: in *Naturata*, Year 1927–28.

Yogananda, Paramahansa: *Autobiography of a Yogi*, Self-Realization Fellowship, Los Angeles 1993.

Zajonc, Arthur: *Catching the Light. The Entwined History of Light and Mind*, Oxford University Press, New York & Oxford 1993.

For more cutting-edge, challenging non-fiction books on current affairs, spirituality, health and the arts, go to:

www.clairviewbooks.com

or e-mail us for a catalogue:

office@clairviewbooks.com